Paths To Knowledge: Innovative Research Methods For Nursing

Barbara Sarter, Editor

Pub. No. 15-2233

National League for Nursing

Copyright © 1988
National League for Nursing
10 Columbus Circle, New York, NY 10019

ISBN 0-88737-415-8

The views expressed in this publication represent the views of the authors and do not necessarily reflect the official views of the National League for Nursing.

Printed in the United States of America

Contents

4. The Ethical Path to Nursing Knowledge

Overview

5. The Intellectual/Interpretive Path to Nursing Knowledge

Overview

Contributors

Barbara J. Bowers, PhD, RN, is Assistant Professor, School of Nursing, University of Wisconsin, Madison, Wisconsin.

Stephenie G. Edgerton, PhD, is Professor of Educational Philosophy, New York University, New York, New York.

Tom Ferentz, MFA, BA, is Photographer, Visual Media Research, University of California, San Francisco, California.

Marsha Fowler, PhD, MSN, RN, is Associate Professor, School of Nursing and Graduate School of Theology, Azusa Pacific University, Azusa, California.

Sarah Fry, PhD, RN, is Associate Professor, School of Nursing, University of Maryland, Baltimore, Maryland.

Betty Highley, MS, RN, FAAN, is Professor, Department of Family Health Care Nursing, and Director, Visual Media Research, University of California, San Francisco, California.

Jan L. Lee, PhD, RN, CS, is Lecturer, School of Nursing, University of California, Los Angeles, California.

Anna Omery, PhD, RN, is Assistant Professor, School of Nursing, University of California, Los Angeles, California.

Francelyn Reeder, PhD, RN, CNM, is Assistant Professor, Associate Faculty of the Center for Human Caring, University of Colorado Health Sciences Center School of Nursing, Denver, Colorado.

Barbara Sarter, PhD, RN, CS, is Assistant Profesor, Department of Nursing, University of Southern California, Los Angeles, California.

Elizabeth Schonwald, MN, RN, is Staff Nurse, Children's Orthopedic Hospital, Seattle, Washington.

Mary Colette Smith, PhD, RN, is Professor, Center for Nursing Research, University of Alabama, Birmingham, Alabama.

Kristen Swanson-Kauffman, PhD, RN, is Research Assistant Professor, Department of Parent and Child Nursing, University of Washington, Seattle, Washington.

Preface

This book is designed to stimulate and challenge a new generation of nurse researchers. It introduces several modes of scholarly inquiry that have been relatively unexplored by nurses, and provides new insights into a number of increasingly popular research methods. The reader will find in these pages a collection of original articles written by leading nurse researchers who have pioneered in the utilization of their respective methodologies. The approach is both scholarly and pragmatic, examining not only the history and philosophical foundations of each method, but discussing such issues as implementation and applications.

The time is ripe for such a book. In their attempts to win acceptance by the academic and scientific communities, early nurse researchers felt impelled to demonstrate competency in traditional experimental research methods. The term "research" became equated with controlled clinical or field studies, with the goal of predicting and manipulating phenomena. In the last decade, the call to broaden the paths to nursing knowledge development has become increasingly strong.

Carper's (1978) landmark article provided a structure to the domain of nursing knowledge that became useful in organizing this book. In addition to empirical ways of knowing, Carper proposed that personal, esthetic, and ethical avenues are necessary for the development of nursing knowledge. The discussions here illustrate all four of these ways of knowing, and present as well a fifth which we may call "intellectual/interpretive." Each of these avenues of knowledge development will be introduced briefly at the beginning of each section of this book.

The anticipated audience for this work ranges from graduate students to mature nursing scholars. Thus, the chapters vary in complexity, depending on the specific method under discussion and the author's depth of analysis. For those who are using this book in the teaching of graduate research courses, it is left to the instructor's discretion to determine appropriate chapters for assignment.

It is with deep respect for and gratitude to the contributors to this book that I present this project. Each contributor has lent herself to this endeavor with enthusiasm and a deep desire to communicate her personal research expertise and experience. I only regret that it is not possible to include in a single volume all of the exciting, pioneering, and scholarly research approaches that are currently under development in our discipline. Perhaps this book will lead to subsequent volumes of a similar nature. A special acknowledgement belongs to Elaine Silverstein, my editor, who has been a constant source of support, advice, and encouragement during this project.

Barbara Sarter

To the Tribe
that still toils
at the Holy Mount Cuchama

Part 1
The Empirical Path
to Nursing Knowledge

The subject matter of empirical research is observable events occurring over a defined span of time. With this broad definition, the research methods included in this section focus on past, present, and future. Historical research explores the events of the past; meta-analysis synthesizes the results of a class of empirical studies; ethnography and grounded theory involve observation of a cultural or social unit of the present; and futures research attempts to anticipate future events in a specified field.

There are numerous empirical research methods not described in these pages; in fact, certain empirical methods comprise the traditional scientific approach to knowledge development. Historical inquiry, ethnography, and grounded theory are inductive approaches to theory development whose purpose is to describe and explain, rather than to predict or control. This goal distinguishes them from other empirical methods of a more experimental nature.

The Historical Method in Nursing

Jan L. Lee

Abraham Lincoln said that "we cannot escape history." Whether we share in the severity of Lincoln's assessment or not, we still cannot evade the responsibility of understanding our past. The need to know and understand accomplishments and trends of the past in order to gain perspective on present and future directions (Kerlinger, 1977) grants historical research its continuing value. Historical research, therefore, has this purpose: to reconstruct the past systematically and objectively by collecting, evaluating, verifying, and synthesizing evidence to establish facts and reach defensible conclusions (Isaac & Michael, 1981).

History itself is defined by Webster's (1984) as: "what has happened in the life or development of a people, country, institution, etc." and as "a systematic account of this, usually in chronological order with an analysis and explanation" (p. 665). As Newton (1965) has observed: "History touches the realm of ideas at more points than almost any other subject" (p. 25). Ashley (1976) has further captured the essence of history: "Facts, events, ideas, institutions and societal trends do not speak for themselves, but must be interpreted by a human mind hard at work trying to analyze the continuity, diversity and change involved in the complex inter-relationships that characterize human history" (p. 30).

Historical research depends on data observed by others, and requires painstaking detective work by historians to analyze the authenticity, accuracy, and significance of source material. As such, it must be rigorous, systematic, and exhaustive (Isaac & Michael, 1981). According to Church (1985), its goal is to establish the knowable truth.

HISTORICAL BACKGROUND

"[History] hath triumphed over time . . ." — Sir Walter Raleigh

Pieces of nursing history have been preserved through ancient writings, such as the Bible, and through art works, inherited from earlier times. But, until recently, historical work in nursing was largely channeled into textbooks, for use in nursing education. These texts not only imparted accepted knowledge but also reflected the profession's view of itself and its relationship to the public (James, 1984).

Examples of widely-used nursing historiography include Nutting and Dock's four-volume *History of Nursing* (1907–1912), Stewart's (1944) *The Education of Nurses*, Roberts' (1954) *American Nursing: History and Interpretation*, Austin's (1957) *History of Nursing Source Book*, and Dolan and Fitzpatrick's (1983), *Nursing in Society: A Historical Perspective*, now in its fifteenth edition. New to the market, and widely acclaimed both for its esthetic approach and its scholarship, is Donahue's (1985) *Nursing, The Finest Art: An Illustrated History*.

Efforts begun in the 1950s have contributed to an enlivening of interest in historical research in nursing. The Yale Survey, funded by the National Institutes of Health, in 1953 began to identify and assess existing research studies in nursing and to bring attention to previously neglected areas. A significant outgrowth of the study was Henderson's four-volume *Nursing Studies Index* (1963–1972). The *Index* provided an annotated guide to the existing, English-speaking, nursing literature from 1900 through 1959. Heralded by James (1984) as "a first-class bibliographic tool" (p. 573), the *Index* was widely accessible, even to inexperienced researchers.

Other nursing periodical indices (*Cummulative Index to Nursing and Allied Health Literature* and the *International Nursing Index*), along with present computer technology which allows for on-line bibliographic searches through the National Library of Medicine, assist the historical nursing researcher in identifying potentially relevant periodicals. Of greater import to nursing historians (those who study history) and historiographers (those who write history), however, has been the development of nursing archive collections. Well-known archives include the Nutting collection at Teachers College in New York and the Nursing Archives, housed in the Mugar Memorial Library in Boston. Other archival collections and nursing history research centers were detailed in the thirty-fifth anniversary issue of *Nursing Research*, which focused on nursing history (Fairman, 1987).

Since 1980, historical research in nursing has been enhanced by the establishment of the American Association for the History of Nursing,

Inc. As initially defined in its "Open Letter" (1987), the mission of this organization is: "to promote historical scholarship and publication in nursing, to help develop centers for preservation and use of historical materials, and to serve as a forum for historical discussion and debate relevant to nursing" (p. 71).

PHILOSOPHICAL ROOTS

". . . history is philosophy teaching by examples." — Henry St. John, Viscount Bolingbroke
    "History repeats itself." — Proverb
    Helen Nahm (1977) has captured the essence of these ageless quotations for nursing:

> I have long been concerned about the need for perspective among nurses in relation to decisions that are made about nursing care, nursing services, and nursing education. I believe such perspective can come only from knowledge of the problems faced by nurses and nursing at particular times in our history and the ability to evaluate the effectiveness of methods used to solve those problems. (p. 218)

THE HISTORICAL METHOD

"The men who make history have not had time to write it." — Metternich
    Teresa Christy (1975), a noted nurse historiographer, has outlined three essential steps in the production of written historical work: (1) the gathering of data, (2) the criticism of the data, and (3) the presentation of facts, interpretations, and conclusions. Recently, the work of revisionists has impacted this process.

Gathering Data

The source materials upon which historians must rely are, in Clubb's (1980) words, "process-produced" (p. 20), that is, the data were not collected, compiled, or preserved with the needs of researchers in mind. In addition, historical research is limited to data and information that have survived the ravages of time.
    Historical data may be collected either from documents (document review) or from persons (oral history). In either case, the historical investigator needs to apply the same framework to data collection, whether in documents or from persons. Thus, an outline for document review

or an interview guide are helpful. The key point is to ask the same questions of each data source.

In gathering data, the historian or historiographer must distinguish between primary and secondary sources. Primary sources are distinguished from secondary sources by the fact that the former give the words of the witnesses or first recorders of an event (Barzun & Graff, 1977), while the latter are all other accounts, at least once removed from actual participation.

However, some documents can be both primary and secondary sources, depending on the purpose of the investigation (Austin, 1958; Kruman, 1985). For instance, in a biography of Lavinia Dock, a passage from a book summarizing Dock's contributions to the nursing profession would be considered a secondary source, whereas in a study of the influence of Lavinia Dock upon the development of the nursing profession, that same passage could be considered a primary source.

Historical Criticism

"In relation to his documents the historian is . . . in the position of 'the single competent witness' " (Barzun & Graff, 1977, p. 141). Critical examination of historical sources, therefore, assumes paramount importance.

Historical criticism involves both external and internal aspects. Stated simply by Clubb (1980), "external criticism is concerned with assessment of the authenticity of sources; internal criticism involves examination of texts to identify error, misrepresentation and inconsistency" (p. 20). Thus, according to Christy (1975), external criticism is concerned with the validity of a document, while internal criticism determines the reliability of the information contained within the document.

As Austin (1958) defines it, external criticism first asks questions about the document itself: "What is it? Is it what it purports to be?" (p. 7). Since the value of a document as a historical source depends to some degree on the writer's motives and the care with which the writer chose the sources, it is important to ascertain how the writer obtained these facts and what effect the writer's motivation may have had on the statements made. Notwithstanding such human variability, external criticism (and validity) is enhanced by the use of primary sources, whenever possible.

The investigator must also be cognizant of the date of the source document as much as of the date of the event under study. Clark (1967) asserts that the most important principle of historical scholarship is the importance of context. In addition, the investigator must ask (Clark, 1967): "Is the document complete? Has it been tampered with or edited?" (p. 62) and, "Through whose hands has this evidence passed?" (p. 81). In sum, the key question is "How reliable is this document?"

Internal criticism seeks to learn the meaning of statements within the document, and to determine their accuracy and trustworthiness. According to Austin (1958), appropriate questions to ask of the source include: "What does this statement mean? In what way does this statement compare with others which I have read on the same subject?" (p. 7).

The investigator's first responsibility is to *understand* the statements in the document (Christy, 1975). This is accomplished by positive internal criticism, which is concerned with ascertaining the *real* versus the *literal* meaning. In positive internal criticism, the investigator must assess the role played by vested interest, the competence of the observer, the opportunity of the writer to have observed the events recorded, and the care taken in recording them (Austin, 1958).

Negative internal criticism, on the other hand, asks that the investigator disbelieve statements until the evidence compels belief (Austin, 1958). Such belief may be designated *fact*, *probability*, or *possibility*, depending on the type and amount of corroborating evidence (Christy, 1975).

Presentation of Facts, Interpretations, and Conclusions

When making inferences and interpretations from the evidence, two questions must be asked (Clark, 1967): "Is the reasoning on which the inference is based correct, and is it the only inference which can be reasonably drawn from the facts?" (p. 57). What history reveals to mankind is not *the cause* of any event but rather *the conditions* attending its emergence. Successive revisions of the past do not cancel each other out but rather add up (Barzun & Graff, 1977) to a more comprehensive understanding of those conditions.

The writing of history is a laborious art, which requires both dedicated precision in adherence to the evidence and creative insight. Kruman (1985) states:

> The research and writing of history is not an impersonal process by which the unvarnished facts present themselves. Instead it is the product of the historian's labor and intelligence acting directly and systematically upon the evidence. (p. 118)

Likewise, Cole (1986) has noted:

> [that] the historian's esthetic of complexity [results in] a subtle and
> balanced portrait based on imaginative mastery of primary sources,
> secondary literature, and voracious reading in related fields. (p. 43)

Impact of the Revisionists

Nurse and other historiographers who have brought a critical analysis
to the study of nursing history have been termed *revisionists* and, simultaneously, *feminists*. One who has painstakingly rewritten a portion of
nursing history deserves the salutation of revisionist. Having contributed
to a new synthesis of the past does not necessarily mean one is a feminist,
however. Although it is hard to imagine analyzing and writing nursing
history without attention to the status of women in America and the
preponderance of women in nursing, a radical feminist perspective is
not required for a legitimate historical critic in nursing. A feminist consciousness would, however, be a common expectation of any nurse historian or historiographer. Also, when revisionist histories become commonly accepted, they will become the new traditional history of nursing,
and the material for future revision.

Meanwhile, as Parsons (1986) has noted:

> With recent additions to women's history and fresh interpretations
> of nursing history, the placement of women at the center of nursing
> history is now possible. Students of nursing, old and new, must direct
> their visions to the influence of Seneca Falls, suffrage, and the Com-
> stock Law. They must ask how nursing influenced events rather than
> how it was influenced by them. Most important, they must claim the
> history that is rightfully theirs, not apologize for it. (p. 274)

Revisionist historiographers of nursing are, indeed, helping nurses re-
claim their history. Ashley's *Hospitals, Paternalism, and the Role of the Nurse*
(1976) introduced a radical feminist viewpoint yet has been criticized
(James, 1984) for its failure to place medical/hospital paternalism within
a meaningful social context, such as in relation to the exploitation of
women in nursing or in relation to the growth of hospitals. Melosh's
(1982) *The Physician's Hand* focused on the work culture of the ordinary
nurse and framed the perennial conflict between worker nurses and
elitist nurse professionalizers. Reverby's (1987) *Ordered to Care* follows in
the tradition of Melosh. For Reverby,

> Nursing as work was transformed in the context of the growth of
> our contemporary health system. It is impossible to retell the story

of nursing without understanding its relationship to the development of medicine. Furthermore, the political economy of the hospital as an institution is as much a part of nursing's history as the political economy of nursing, in turn, is integral to the history of the hospital and of medicine. (p. 2)

Recent journal articles have also echoed a revisionist theme. Representative cases are the work of Lovell (1980), Parsons (1986), and Wagner (1980).

POTENTIAL PROBLEMS IN HISTORICAL RESEARCH

"God cannot alter the past, but historians can." — Samuel Butler

Many problems may arise in implementing historical research. Common difficulties include: (1) lack of problem clarity, (2) lack of theoretical framework, (3) access to source data, (4) condition of source data, (5) difficulty staying focused, (6) imprecise documentation, (7) neglect of context, (8) the creative challenge, and (9) research preparation.

Lack of Problem Clarity

An unclear statement of the problem at hand will usually cause confusion regarding data collection. An imprecise problem formulation, coupled with actual conceptual imprecision, will negatively impact validity and reliability. As noted earlier, lack of problem clarity will also negatively impact generalizability.

Lack of Theoretical Framework

Because it is essential to ground the study and provide a consistent approach to the data, a theoretical framework is an integral part of any research endeavor. This is especially true of historical research, where the investigator is intimately involved in the selection, identification, abstraction, and interpretation of data by intellectual means rather than by statistical or other measuring devices. For example, in a study of the emergence of the concept, patient/client agency, in the nursing literature 1900–1986, this author utilized the chronological development of nursing knowledge (after Meleis, 1985) as an appropriate theoretical framework. Any lack or weakness in the theoretical framework will also contribute to confusion and imprecision in data collection and interpretation.

Access to Source Data

Data needed for a particular study may be isolated in one or more selected locations distant from the investigator. Unless time and money are available to allow for travel to locate source data, the investigator may decide to modify the research problem in light of the data more readily available.

Whenever historical study is proposed, it is important for the investigator to weigh the fragility of the source versus the importance of the study at hand. This process may assist in problem clarification. It will also be instrumental in helping to verify scholarly intent and credentials as one seeks official entree to protected sources. Obviously, these comments apply equally well to persons as to source documents.

Condition of Source Data

Problems may result from poor preservation of source documents, from poor quality photocopies or facsimiles of original documents, or from the altered cognition of elderly or ill source persons. The investigator must be cognizant of the types of source data and consequently make a reasoned decision as to which to use. No matter the choice, the investigator must identify limitations in the sources chosen. For instance, reproductions of early volumes of the *American Journal of Nursing* are indeed reproduced word for word in article and editorial content. Advertisements, however, have been eliminated. Since valuable clues to social, economic, and technologic trends of the time can be gleaned through advertisements, their absence is a loss that needs to be acknowledged.

Difficulty Staying Focused

To accomplish historical research in an efficient yet meaningful way, one must, while maintaining focus on the described goal, also allow for openness to related issues and insights. However, becoming mired in peripheral issues which distract from the original intent of the study can prove dangerous to appropriate outcomes. In reality, historical studies do sometimes take important detours. Therefore, it is important to maintain focus while reassessing periodically the character of the focus maintained.

Imprecise Documentation

Imprecise documentation may be a function of the data source itself; or, it may be a function of the investigator's data collection procedures.

As previously noted, a form can be useful in increasing the consistency of data collected. Such a form may also supply clues important to recording information necessary for subsequent citations, such as a complete journal reference or the date, time, and location of an interview. Investigator aids, such as data collection forms, an outline of data collection procedures, or an oral history guide can increase both reliability and validity of study conclusions.

Neglect of Context

As discussed above, no historical person, event, or pattern can be analyzed in isolation, out of context. Because of this, revisionist historians and historiographers continue to demand that all historical researchers account for context. In other words, to adequately address a historical problem one must attend to appropriate surrounding forces. For nursing, such contextual forces may include social, technologic, environmental, economic, and political trends.

The Creative Challenge

Intellectual analysis, the conceptual molding that eventually results in a re-formation of data, is the greatest challenge of historical research. This re-formation may or may not represent actual revision. It may or may not reinforce the traditional conceptualization of the period under study, as well. What it most certainly will have done, however, is to cause a new synthesis by an open mind. Given that that mind is disciplined, consistent, and logical, and that the data analyzed were valid and reliable, the conclusions drawn are amenable to generalization across similar data, persons, or events in similar contexts.

Researcher Preparation

Researcher preparation is an especially critical element in the historical research process, due to the direct effect of the investigator upon the data and vice versa. Like any research endeavor, investigators preparing to take on historical research must experience the process, do the research, face the challenges, solve the problems, and complete the intellectual exercise.

Several suggestions may assist the researcher new to the historical method in producing a more credible product. First, read widely in the historical literature, both within, and outside of, nursing. Focus on both the methodology and the narrative, thereby gaining a healthy appreciation for both the science of historical criticism and the art of historical storytelling. Second, hone the problem into a clear, unambiguous statement or question. Third, select an applicable theoretical framework that will serve to ground the project and to give direction. Fourth, build safeguards into the data collection process to increase validity, reliability, and generalizability. Fifth, remember the importance of context. If at all possible, utilize interdisciplinary peers for critique at various stages of the research endeavor. Sixth, recognize the inevitability of investigator bias. Try to suspend these biases. Seventh, release creative powers through such techniques as brainstorming and imagery to envision a reality, but one *which comes from the data.*

The writing of a historical narrative, however, is something else, of another order entirely. And nothing, except the writing itself, can prepare the researcher for this task. Expected capacities, such as word finding, breadth of vocabulary, and grammar and syntax skills, are necessary, but certainly not sufficient. What must be present beyond the mechanics of written communications is the intellectual capacity to conceptualize and the creative freedom to merge and meld old and new concepts and events in old and new ways. The experience of writing a historical study is the experience of creating a new whole, which truly is more than the sum of its parts.

ROLE OF HISTORICAL METHOD IN THEORY DEVELOPMENT AND TESTING

"Human history is in essence a history of ideas." — Herbert George Wells

The historical method has three major roles in relation to theory development and testing. First, it is useful in tracing the chronology of knowledge development in nursing. Second, with its context-dependent criteria, it is helpful in clarifying the antecedent factors, philosophical underpinnings, and resulting products that have evolved in the field of nursing theory development. Third, tenets of the historical method can be indirectly employed in present-day theory testing studies to ascertain to what degree the theory as utilized in the present study is consistent with the theory as presented traditionally. Discrepancies between traditional (historical) depictions and the present (reformed or revisionist) depiction may illustrate misunderstanding, modifications, or evolution.

CONCLUSION

The continual need to reexamine and reexplore the past in order to better understand the present and to better prepare for the future necessitates the development of new nurse historians and historiographers. This chapter has explored in brief the use of the historical method in nursing as a reputable research endeavor, with a long and varied history. Tenets of the historical method were reviewed, potential problems inherent in the historical method were explored, and the role of the historical method in theory development and testing was described.

REFERENCES

An open letter to our colleagues in nursing and history. (1987). *Nursing Research, 36,* 71.

Ashley, J. A. (1976). *Hospitals, paternalism, and the role of the nurse.* New York: Teachers College Press.

Ashley, J. A. (1978). Foundations for scholarship: Historical research in nursing. *Advances in Nursing Science, 1*(1), 25–36.

Austin, A. L. (1957). *History of nursing source book.* New York: G.P. Putnam's Sons.

Austin, A. L. (1958). The historical method in nursing. *Nursing Research, 7*(1), 4–10.

Barzun, J., & Graff, H. F. (1977). *The modern researcher* (3rd ed.). New York: Harcourt Brace Jovanovich.

Christy, T. E. (1975). The methodology of historical research: A brief introduction. *Nursing Research, 24,* 189–192.

Church, O. M. (1985). New knowledge from old truths: Problems and promises of historical inquiry in nursing. In J. C. McCloskey & H. K. Grace (Eds.), *Current issues in nursing* (2nd ed.). Boston: Blackwell Scientific Publications.

Clark, G. K. (1967) *The critical historian.* New York: Basic Books.

Clubb, J. M. (1980). The new quantitative history: Social science or old wine in new bottles? In J. M. Clubb, & E.K. Scheuch (Eds.), *Historical social research: The use of historical and process-produced data.* Stuttgart, Germany: Ernst Klett.

Cole, T. R. (1986). Reviews: When conservative medicine triumphed and feminist values failed. *Hastings Center Report, 16,* 43–45.

Dolan, J. A., & Fitzpatrick, M.L. (1983). *Nursing in society: A historical perspective* (15th ed.). Philadelphia: W. B. Saunders.

Donahue, M. P. (1985). *Nursing, the finest art: An illustrated history.* St. Louis: C. V. Mosby.

Fairman, J. A. (1987). Sources and references for research in nursing history. *Nursing Research, 36,* 56–59.

Henderson, V. (1963–1972). *Nursing studies index: Volumes I-IV.* Philadelphia: Lippincott.

Isaac, S., & Michael, W. B. (1981). *Handbook in research and evaluation* (2nd ed.). San Diego, CA: Edits Publishers.

James, J. W. (1984). Writing and rewriting nursing history: A review essay. *Bulletin of the History of Medicine, 58,* 568–584.

Kerlinger, F. N. (1973). *Foundations of behavioral research* (2nd ed.). New York: Holt, Rinehart.

Kruman, M. W. (1985). Historical method: Implications for nursing research. In M. Leininger (Ed.), *Qualitative research methods in nursing.* Orlando, FL: Grune & Stratton.

Lovell, M. C. (1980). The politics of medical deception: Challenging the trajectory of history. *Advances in Nursing Science, 2*(3), 73–86.

Meleis, A. I. (1985). *Theoretical nursing: Development and progress.* Philadelphia: Lippincott.

Melosh, B. (1982). *The physician's hand: Work culture and conflict in American nursing.* Philadelphia: Temple University Press.

Nahm, H. (1977). Letters: Nursing's history. *Nursing Research, 25,* 218.

Newton, M. E. (1965). The case for historical research. *Nursing Research, 14*(1), 20–26.

Nutting, M.A., & Dock, L. L. (1907–1912). *History of nursing: Volumes I-IV.* New York: G. P. Putnam's Sons.

Parsons, M. (1986). The profession in a class by itself. *Nursing Outlook, 34,* 270–275.

Reverby, S. M. (1987). *Ordered to care: The dilemma of American Nursing. 1850–1945.* New York: Cambridge University Press.

Roberts, M. M. (1954). *American nursing: History and interpretation.* New York: Macmillan.

Stewart, I. M. (1944). *The education of nurses.* New York: Macmillan.

Wagner, D. (1980). The proletarianization of nursing in the United States, 1932–1946. *International Journal of Health Services, 10,* 190–271.

Webster's new world dictionary (2nd College ed.). (1984). New York: Simon & Schuster.

Ethnography

Anna Omery

What are the health beliefs of Navaho Native Americans in regard to exercise? What is the response of women who were born in the Middle East to abdominal surgery? What do nurses who have worked only in critical care expect from the nurse–physician relationship? Is this expectation different for the nurse who has worked exclusively in a psychiatric setting? These are a few of the research questions that need to be answered if nursing's practice is to be effectual. The research method that will best answer these questions is ethnography.

Ethnography is the research method committed to describing the social and cultural worlds of a particular group (Emerson, 1983). It provides an empirical description of the phenomenon of interest from a specific cultural or societal focus. This description includes the knowledge, behaviors, beliefs, and meanings that are integral to that culture or society.

The scope of ethnography can be broad, such as the study of a complex society, which is then considered as *macroethnography*. Or, the scope can be limited to a subunit of a single institution, such as a nursing unit, which is then considered *microethnography*.

Whatever the scope, the central aim of ethnography is to describe another way of life from the "native point of view" (Spradley, 1980). It seeks to discover the cultural or social knowledge that people use to organize their behavior and understand their life experiences (Germain, 1986). As such, ethnography is the disciplined study of what the world is like to the people who have always lived in that world.

When nurse researchers wish to understand some actual or potential human response to illness, that is, some health belief or practice, from a specific cultural or social perspective, they should employ ethnography.

17

For example, a nurse researcher whose area of interest or practice is health care of recent immigrants from Lebanon might wish to describe the response to surgery that is culturally specific to that population. Nurses could then design interventions appropriate to those culturally specific responses which would not conflict with any of the world views of the individuals for whom they provide care.

Historical Background

While most civilizations since at least the times of the Greeks have observed their sister cultures in some systematic fashion, as a modern research method, ethnography finds its roots in the traditions of cultural anthropology and American sociology (Kirk & Miller, 1986).

Generally credited with the establishment of the profession of cultural anthropology, Franz Boaz, in his studies at Columbia at the turn of the last century, underscored the necessity of direct investigation. Against the "armchair habits" of his peers, for whom ethnography was considered an intellectual diversion and scholarly pursuit, he promoted the invaluable method of data collection from the field. He understood that unless the ethnographer was there and trained to observe accurately, data, to say nothing of context, would remain second hand and appropriately suspect.

Bronislaw Malinowski further developed the research process that was to become ethnography. A Polish citizen, Malinowski was detained in the South Pacific by the British government during World War I. He used the opportunity to study several of the indigenous populations. During these studies, he also emphasized accurate data collection. In addition, he further expanded ethnography to include the necessary elements of analysis and interpretation of the data collected from the field.

American Sociology, specifically the Chicago School of the 1920s and 1930s, also made significant contributions to ethnography. During those years, participant observation as a data collection technique was a special area of concern. It was at Chicago that this technique was sophisticated to meet enhanced criteria for validity.

Each of these advances chronologically overlapped the other; an advance in one resulted in refinement in the other two. As a result of these advances, a method was created which promoted professional, scientific findings or descriptions of cultures and societies.

PHILOSOPHICAL ROOTS/EPISTEMOLOGICAL ASSUMPTIONS

As a qualitative method, ethnography shares several epistemological assumptions with all other qualitative research methods. The most important of these are the emphasis on descriptive understanding and the inclusion of all data.

For most qualitative as opposed to quantitative research methods, the goal is *understanding*. However, there is no guarantee from any qualitative method that it will provide *explanation*, *verification*, *prediction* or *control*. These, rather, are the goals of quantitative research designs. On the other hand, qualitative methods do provide a description of the phenomenon of interest with information sufficient to comprehend or perceive that phenomenon. The degree of abstraction of that perception, whether the product is simple description or formal theory, remains a function of the specific qualitative method.

Another assumption that is fundamental to qualitative methods is the belief that all data should and will be included in data collection and anaylsis. There is no such thing as an "outlier" for any qualitative method. All data are important. It is not left up to the investigator to determine which data are germane or relevant. Outside rules or standards do not function to exclude findings. The intent is the discovery of the nature of the phenomenon as experienced by those who participate in the phenomenon. As such, all data related to the subject under investigation is suitable for collection and appropriate for inclusion at the time of analysis.

In addition to these generic assumptions, ethnography has several epistemological suppositions that are specific to itself. The most important of these suppositions are not contentious for those who employ ethnography. However, there are other epistemological postulates which are contentious for some ethnographers.

Robertson and Boyle (1984) point out that essentially all ethnographers share an epistemological conviction that human behavior can only be understood within the context in which it occurs. Behavior is believed to be holistic or ecological, that is, it can only be understood within its functional, cultural, or societal system (Knapp, 1979). As a consequence, there is an emphasis on conducting ethnographic studies in the natural setting: the setting where the phenomenon under investigation actually occurs. Traditionally, these natural settings have been conceptualized as distant and exotic places in Africa or Polynesia. Functionally, they could include any cultural setting; for example, a medical-surgical nursing unit.

More problematic are the polarized epistemological presumptions related to the *emic* or *etic* orientation. Both of these terms denote a general orientation of what constitutes reality in ethnographic research. Extreme adherence to one or the other results in the choice of a mutually exclusive research approach (Monrey & Luthans, 1984).

When a researcher operates from an emic approach, the researcher believes that knowledge is acquired through a discernment of the informant's view of reality. Therefore, understanding of behavior can only be accomplished when the researcher appreciates or comprehends the behavior according to the perception and interpretations of those engaging in that behavior. The researcher will use an approach which seeks to explain how the study population constructs reality in its own terms (Morey & Luthrans, 1984; Pelto & Pelto, 1978; Robertson & Boyle,1984; Schartz & Jacobs, 1979).

The ethnographer operating from an emic perspective will examine the language of the culture, learn the organizing frameworks, and describe the cultural perception of reality from the viewpoint of a member of that culture. It requires the researcher to intensively enter the informant's world or life view including the purpose, meanings, and beliefs of that view. By meeting this requirement, the ethnographer goes beyond knowledge to an understanding of the culture and its practices (Kay & Evaneshko, 1982). When an ethnographer operates from an emic perspective, he or she believes that "between the actor and observer, it is the actor who is better able to know his own inner state" (Harris, 1968).

In contrast, the etic orientation designates a researcher who seeks to organize the subjects' world or culture according to the categories or theoretical perspectives of ethnography. Extreme adherents of this approach believe that the researcher is the most appropriate adjudicator of the adequacy of the final description or understanding. As a result, more significance is placed on the informant's observed behavior than is placed on that person's cognitive state. The informant's opinion may be interesting, but it is not necessarily relevant (Harris, 1979).

As with most extremes, strict adherence to either the emic or etic orientation is problematic. The exclusive use of either results in potential loss of data and, therefore, of a comprehensive understanding of the living world under investigation. To resolve such difficulties, most ethnographers employ an eclectic research style which integrates both epistomological presuppositions (Punch, 1985). Such an eclectic, integrative style results in an extensive account of the phenomena being studied (Pelto & Pelto, 1978).

PREPARATION OF THE RESEARCHER

How does a researcher "do" ethnography?

The first nurse ethnographers were those that studied for advanced degrees in the disciplines of cultural anthropology and sociology. In addition to formal courses on the process of ethnography, these nurses often were apprenticed to a master ethnographer whose focus was usually cross-cultural fieldwork. Indeed, and as Wolcott (1975) states, there are those who continue to feel that this combination of didactic and apprenticeship is still the most appropriate way to gain competence in ethnography.

Current preparation in ethnography by nurse researchers continues for many in those other disciplines. Many other nurse researchers are, however, learning this non-traditional research process as they study for advanced degrees in their own discipline of nursing. This preparation may come from those nurses who studied in other fields and returned to share their expertise in nursing. Or, it may come from a growing group of nurses who have been exposed to ethnography as a part of their advanced study in nursing.

In addition to courses in ethnography, the researcher who is contemplating a research project using this method should have had some exposure to research ethics. While it is helpful for any study, including an ethnographic one, to be reviewed by an institutional or human subjects review committee, the investigator should not expect that review or any forms or procedures that are the result of that review to finalize ethical considerations related to that study.

The researcher who expects to complete an ethnographic study should be prepared to face difficult questions. Should the participant observer also participate; if so, to what extent? What will the investigator's response be if it becomes apparent that illegal activities are being observed? Consideration of these and other pertinent questions should take place before the beginning of any data collection (Barnes, 1970; Punch, 1985).

Exposure to such concerns could come from formal courses in research ethics. Exposure also could come from discussions in support groups that consist of other ethnographic or qualitative researchers. However exposure does occur, discussions concerning ethical issues should include: the identification of ways to safeguard informants' rights, interest, and sensitivities; when and how to communicate research objectives and findings; and strategies for protecting the privacy of the informants. In all cases, emphasis should be on how not to exploit the informant who has agreed to let the investigator be a part of his or her world.

Establishing or identifying a support group will also be of benefit for many other issues. Ethnography is often lonely. It can involve physical, psychological, and emotional stress (Germain, 1986). During such times, a support group may become a critical factor toward the successful conclusion of the study. It may even become the foremost factor in supporting the investigator toward that conclusion.

In addition to formal or informal preparation, there are several requirements that any investigator should satisfy related to personal likes and dislikes prior to the initiation of any ethnographic study. Germain (1985) has identified several of these criteria for consideration. Ethnographers should like to learn, especially about new cultures. They should like to collect and process their own data. They should be willing and able to report the findings in a narrative as opposed to statistical format. In addition, they should be prepared to be comfortable with some degree of potential culture shock and the possibility of being constantly faced with ambiguity. Obviously, the ethnographer should be able to build trusting relationships with the members of the culture under investigation. The researcher may conclude that he or she is not comfortable or able to meet these requirements. In that case, the research project is probably best served by establishing liaison with another researcher who does feel comfortable in meeting those considerations.

THE RESEARCH PROCESS

Ethnography is participating, overtly or covertly, in people's lives for an extended period. It is watching what is happening, listening to what is being said. It is asking questions or collecting whatever data is available to throw light on or understand the issue or practice under investigation. It is also analyzing and organizing that data in a written narrative that describes that issue or practice.

The general research process reported here follows the steps identified by Spradley (1979, 1980). The reader is reminded that in the identification of any stepwise progression for any research method, the division into steps is often arbitrary, reflecting either the education or idiosyncracies of the author. The content of any specific research process should, however, be consistent across authors. The content of the steps identified in this discussion is consistent with the content of the process identified by other ethnographers, including Germain (1985) and Hammersley and Atkinson (1983).

Spradley (1979, 1980) describes ethnography as a research cycle consisting of six steps. The six steps are:

1. Selecting an ethnographic project.
2. Asking ethnographic questions.
3. Collecting ethnographic data.
4. Making an ethnographic record.
5. Analyzing ethnographic data.
6. Writing an ethnography.

Ethnography also implicates a research cycle in that the writing of the findings generates new ethnographic projects. As the researcher selects one of these projects, he or she begins anew the research process of ethnography.

Step One: Selecting an Ethnographic Project

The process of selecting an ethnographic project is both the easiest and most difficult step in the research cycle. The selection process is easy in that the researcher is lead to ethnography only if, by way of the research question, he or she seeks to describe or understand a particular culture or subculture. If the purpose of the research is concept description or description of a basic sociological process, then ethnography is not the appropriate research method. Rather, the researcher should explore phenomenology and grounded theory methods.

However, the selection of an ethnographic project is difficult in that several other factors must be considered before one can move to the next step in the research process, including: the scope of the project, the identification of the setting, and gaining access to the setting.

As indicated earlier, the scope of an ethnographic project can range along a continuum from macro to microethnography. The continuum extends from the description of complex societies at the macro extreme to description of a single social situation at the micro extreme. Prior to entry into data collection, the investigator must determine the scope of the investigation that he or she wishes to undertake. If the investigator(s) fails to determine the scope of the project before beginning data analysis, they run the risk of collecting data that is either too specific to a subculture of the whole that they wish to understand or too inexplicit to describe the small unit or subculture that they wish to delineate.

The investigator also must consider that scope may be predetermined by external factors. These factors may include limited access to the field for data collection, limited resources, such as time or money, or ethical or legal considerations.

Once the scope of the research setting has been determined, the researcher must consider which settings are appropriate for data collection. For example, nurses may be interested in examining subcultures related to health in their own society. The selection of the ethnographic project then should include which specific settings must be addressed to describe the situation holistically. Consider an ethnographer who wishes to examine how elderly diabetic clients maintain their prescribed dietary regime. Should the observations or interviews take place only in the nutritionist's office? Should data collection be limited to the subjects' homes? Should the settings include the patient teaching activities in the acute hospital or doctor's office? Or, should all of these settings be included in the final description?

Finally, the researcher must consider gaining access during the selection of the project. Several levels of clearance or consent may be required before the ethnographer can enter the field. Such factors as frequency and hours of coming and going, the means of identification of the ethnographer, permission to use recording devices, determination of what data sources or fields are absolutely off limits, and to what degree the investigator will participate in the setting must be established in advance so far as possible (Germain, 1985).

Once the project has been selected, the researcher must document each of the decisions with detail. These details may become necessary as the investigator seeks to determine several months or sites later the rationale for a specific decision. Also, it will aid the investigator in writing up the ethnography at the completion of the research cycle.

Step Two: Asking Ethnographic Questions

Ethnographic fieldwork begins when the investigator starts to ask questions. In traditional research, the questions asked by the researcher come from a preselected list determined by a guiding conceptual or theoretical framework. In ethnography, the questions and answers must come from the specific culture or society being questioned. The task of the ethnographer is to discover questions that seek relationships that are meaningful to participants of the culture under study (Spradley, 1980). All ethnography begins with broad descriptive questions (What are these people doing here? What is the nature of this setting?). Later, after analyzing the initial data, the questions will become more specific and focused.

Step Three: Collecting Ethnographic Data

Whereas Step Two is operationalized when one starts asking questions, Step Three is operationalized through participant observation. Step Two may precede Step Three. Or, the ethnographer may find the two steps are operationalized concurrently.

In participant observation, the ethnographer attempts to enter the subculture by participating in a manner that induces as little change as possible (Germain, 1985). The ethnographer observes the activities of the participants, the physical characteristics of the situation, and what it feels like to be a part of the site (Spradley, 1980). The investigator begins by making broad descriptive observations, then he or she starts to focus those observations. Finally, the investigator concludes the data collection with selective observations that confirm the description or understanding being developed.

Junker (1960) describes a range of participant observation. He notes that during the course of data collection the investigator might use all of the four types of participant observation, which are:

1. Complete Observer. In this type, the investigator may be visible, but does not interact with those being observed. Indeed, the observation may even be covert.

2. Observer-as-Participant. In this type, the role of the observer is publicly known at the onset. While the investigator may participate, if necessary, the role is primarily focused on observation.

3. Participant-as-Observer. In this type, the observer activities are subordinated to activities as participant. Participants or informants are aware, however, that the investigator is also an observer collecting data.

4. Complete Participant. In this type, the participant-observer's roles as observer are deliberately and intentionally concealed. Informants are unaware that they are being observed and data collected.

In today's research environment, the two extreme types, Complete Observer and Complete Participant, may by problematic for the researcher to assume. These roles, if covert, could be considered unethical as they violate the informed consent of the subjects.

Step Four: Making an Ethnographic Record

This step is the bridge between data collection and data analysis. During this step, the investigator creates the ethnographic notebook. This notebook consists of observational, methodological, and theoretical notes. Observational notes are the actual details or descriptors from the field. Methodological notes are details reminding the investigator where and how he or she gathered the data. Theoretical notes are initial or preliminary perceptions concerning the final description or understanding.

The investigator should review the ethnographic notebook at least once daily (and preferably more often) during data collection. The investigator should also transcribe all notes at the end of each day. The typed field notes should be double spaced with wide margins to assist in the coding of data.

The time for processing field notes far accedes the time for data collection. Careful processing will, however, assist the investigator by guiding further data collection and in manipulating the data during analysis.

Step Five: Analyzing Ethnographic Data

Ethnographic analysis is the process of inductively identifying patterns or themes from data as a result of logical analysis. When the investigator has extracted all thematic or pattern categories from the data, he or she can establish their relationships in regard to the culture under study as a whole.

This process of comparing, contrasting, analyzing, and synthesizing takes time and considerable mental effort. However, this should not prevent the investigator from recording each step in the process of analysis. Systematic recording may be shared in the writing of the ethnography or it may be used by the investigator in further data collection for verification of the final description.

The cycle of collection, management, and analysis of data has been described sequentially. In reality, Steps Two through Five will often occur concurrently. The cycle continues until the investigator achieves a comprehensive and exhaustive description of the culture.

Step Six: Writing an Ethnography

This last, major task can also lead to new questions and ethnographic projects. Certainly, it can force the investigator back into the field to collect more data. Spradley (1980) notes that this step is like climbing a very tall tree to view the forest from an elevated perspective. It provides the broad scope, outlines the tasks completed, and suggests direction to future tasks or projects.

Ethnography is usually reported in the style of literal narrative, which should enhance the essence and nuances of the culture or society described. The narrative format also allows the reader to progress from concrete to abstract when that is required. For example, while findings may be limited to constructed taxonomies of descriptors, findings may, however, progress to highly abstract descriptions or understandings.

In the final narrative, the ethnographer may choose to organize the narrative as a natural history, which may be chronological or spacial in nature. The ethnographer may also choose to organize the report around significant themes.

The specific organization of the report may reflect the background of the investigator. The organization or style may also be affected by the intended audience. The ethnographer may, for example, write in one manner if the intended audience is a group of fellow ethnographers, and in another style if the audience is a group of researchers unfamiliar with qualitative research.

Issues of Validity, Reliability, and Generalizability

What are some of the researcher's concerns as they implement the method?

The extent to which issues of validity, reliability, and generalizability will be of concern to a researcher is, to a certain degree, a function of the epistemological standpoint of that researcher. Validity, reliability, and generalizability were developed as indicators of the robustness of certain types of research designs or instruments traditionally associated with a deductive and positivistic view of science. This view depicts the goal of science as the development of theory that is capable of prediction and control. However, ethnography is associated with an alternate inductive view of science. This view depicts the goal of ethnography as description and understanding. There are researchers committed to this alternate view who also feel that these indicators are appropriate only for use by the deductive science for which they were developed. On the other hand, different researchers feel that the indicators are appropriate for all views of science. It is in the interpretation and implementation of the indicators that concerns must be addressed (Kirk & Miller, 1986).

Ethnographers who reject validity, reliability, and generalizability are as concerned about the scientific merit of their research as any other scientist. They only reject such indicators as the criteria for that merit. Agar (1986), for example, argues that ethnography is a different research style with a different purpose: description. Therefore, it should not be critiqued using criteria developed for the deductive purpose of prediction and control. However, these researchers have failed to identify alternate criteria for evaluating merit which are acceptable to the scientific community, even if one limits that community to only those researchers comfortable with qualitative research.

Still other ethnographers advocate a third, compromise position: the use of one or more of the criteria, but only after they have been adjusted to meet the demands of the alternative epistemological standpoint.

For these ethnographers, validity is how accurately the researcher charts the observed reality and then delineates that reality in the written report (Germain, 1986). Threats to validity include inaccurate or incomplete observations and self-serving error or bias. These threats may be the result of the particular spatial location of the observer, the social skewing of reported opinion, or the particular cultural or societal alignment of the observer (Loftland & Loftland, 1984). Validity is achieved through a lengthy stay in the culture being observed, extensive and intensive data collection, verification of the observations, and the narrative report of the findings with as many cultural informants as possible.

Reliability is more troublesome for the ethnographer. One cannot replicate an ethnography. Therefore, reliability entails maximizing the consistency of both the sources of data, including informants and researcher, and the methods of data collection (Germain, 1986). Consistency of informant data can be established with inter-informant reliability (Pelto & Pelto, 1978). Researcher consistency can be authenticated by having two or more observers observe and record the same event. Collecting data from a variety of sources can also aid in reliability (Robertson & Boyle, 1984).

For ethnography, generalizability or external validity is limited to all those sharing the same culture or participating in the same kinds of activities (Knapp, 1979). While the ideographic focus and inductive logic of ethnography does not match the penchant of researchers for generalizable results based on nomothetic research knowledge and deductive logic, the explicit and worthwhile insights generated may be more profound and purposeful than generalizable findings from a study of variables in isolation from meaningful context (Germain, 1986; Knapp, 1979).

POTENTIAL PROBLEMS IN IMPLEMENTATION

Spradley (1980) identifies four recurring problem areas in implementation: fieldwork, conceptual, analysis, and writing problems. Fieldwork problems include cancelled appointments, failure to gain access to the most desired field for data collection, unwillingness to answer questions, suspicion, and failure to gain rapport. Conceptual problems are usually the result of a lack of understanding of fundamental concepts related to doing ethnography. Analysis problems come from not knowing what to do with the raw information gathered from participant observation. Writing problems include organizing the final report and knowing what to include as well as how to go about the task of writing.

With careful preparation, the ethnographer can decrease the frequency and magnitude of these problems. By seeking out the expertise of the more experienced researcher and networking with a support group, the researcher can anticipate many of the problems in the field. By this process, the researcher can either prevent problems altogether or facilitate the use of corrective strategies or tactics should specific problems arise.

Every ethnographer should remember, however, that each ethnography is unique—some problems may not be amenable to anticipation; some corrective strategies may not work in the new setting. The key to success in overcoming such problems is to remain flexible, creative, and sagacious.

HOW CAN ETHNOGRAPHY INFLUENCE THE DEVELOPMENT OR TESTING OF THEORY?

Most ethnographers agree that their major contribution to other disciplines is in the development of new descriptive theory. Such theories may reflect cultural knowledge, behaviors, or meanings.

Such theories are the result of first-hand contact with the people and settings concerned and are developed from the observed life experiences of the subjects under study. As such, they are less prone to errors of conceptual omission or commission than are those theories which are the product of the "armchair theorist."

It is important, however, for the budding theorist to keep in mind that the type of theory developed from an ethnography has, as its goal, description and understanding. It will not necessarily result in the development of a highly abstract predictive theory to be used in explication of cause and effect relationships.

The use of ethnography for theory testing is not as well established. However, if one considers the documentation of theoretical concepts and their relationships to theory testing, then there is every reason for ethnography to accomplish that task, as well. Indeed, Kirk and Miller (1986) feel that the use of qualitative methods, such as ethnography, for that purpose have been ignored. Conceivably, as a result of that disregard some theory may not be as well conceptualized or authenticated as would otherwise be possible.

CONCLUSION

Because nursing is a practice discipline, its knowledge or theory base needs to be broad enough to allow comprehensive nursing care to all possible patients, no matter their background. This type of care is only possible when nurses have some notion of the salient cultural factors related to health and illness. Ethnographic nursing research can provide much needed data not only for nursing, but for all disciplines that wish to provide health care to patients from diverse cultural experiences.

REFERENCES

Agar, M. (1986). *Speaking of ethnography*. Beverly Hills: Sage Publications.

Barnes, J. A. (1970). Some ethical problems in modern fieldwork. In W. Filstead (Ed.), *Qualitative methodology*. Chicago: Markum, Inc.

Emerson, R. M. (1983). *Contemporary field research*. Boston: Little Brown and Co.

Germain, C. (1986). Ethnography: The method. In P. Munhall & C. Oiler (Eds.), *Nursing research: A qualitative perspective*. Norwalk: Appleton-Century-Crofts.

Hammersley, M., & Atkinson, P. (1983). *Ethnography: Principles in practice*. New York: Tavistock Publications.

Harris, M. (1968). *The rise of anthropological theory*. New York: Thomas Y. Crowell Publications.

Harris, M. (1979). *Cultural materialism: The struggle for a science of culture*. New York: Random House.

Junker, B. (1960). *Field work*. Chicago: University of Chicago Press.

Kay, M. A., & Evanenshko, V. (1982). The ethnoscience research technique. *Western Journal of Nursing Research, 4*, 49–64.

Kirk, J., & Miller, M. (1986). *Reliability and validity in qualitative research*. Beverly Hills: Sage Publications.

Knapp, M. S. (1979). Ethnographic contributions to evaluation research. In T. D. Cook, & C. S. Reichardt (Eds.), *Qualitative and quantitative methods in evaluation research*. Beverly Hills: Sage Publications.

Loftland, J., & Loftland, L. (1984). *Analyzing social settings* (2nd ed.). Belmont: Wadsworth Publishing Co.

Monrey, N., & Luthans, F. (1984). An emic perspective and ethnoscience methods for organizational research. *Academy of Management Review*, *9*(1), 27–36.

Pelto, P., & Pelto, G. (1978). *Anthropological research: The structure of inquiry.* New York: Cambridge University Press.

Punch, M. (1985). *The politics and ethics of fieldwork.* Beverly Hills: Sage Publications.

Robertson, M., & Boyle, J. (1984). Ethnography: Contributions to nursing research. *Journal of Advanced Nursing*, *9*, 43–49.

Schartz, H., & Jacobs, H. (1979). *Qualitative sociology: A method to the madness.* New York: The Free Press.

Spradley, J. (1979). *The ethnographic interview.* New York: Holt, Rhinehart, and Winston.

Spradley, J. (1980). *Participant observation.* New York: Holt, Rhinehart, and Winston.

Wolcott, H. F. (1975). Criteria for an ethnographic approach to research in schools. *Human Organization*, *34*, 114–118.

Grounded Theory

Barbara J. Bowers

The intellectual roots of the grounded theory method can be traced directly to the Chicago School of Sociology. The Chicago School, as it has come to be known, refers to the social psychology of symbolic interactionism and related research methods developed at the University of Chicago during the period between 1920 and 1950.[1]

Symbolic interactionism was in part a reaction against the grand functionalist theories of social action which dominated sociological thought during the mid-nineteenth century. Functionalism, elaborated largely by Talcott Parsons, Robert Merton, and other functionalists, was virtually synonymous with sociological theory at the time (Friedrichs, 1972; Coser, 1977; Camic, 1987; Gouldner, 1970). The Chicago School, which was most influential during the 1920s, represented the first major challenge to the hegemonic status of functionalist theory (Friedrichs, 1972).

FUNCTIONALISM

Because symbolic interactionism differs significantly from functionalism and because many nursing theories are informed by functionalist theory, a brief overview of the theory can provide a useful starting place for discussion.[2] Functionalism can be characterized as a theoretical position that the (social) world exists as a whole unit or system which is comprised of interrelated, functioning parts. Functionalism is, according to Gouldner (1970), "an unshakable metaphysical conviction: that the world is one" (p. 199). The focus of functionalist analysis or theorizing is on the system as a whole, the smoothness of its overall functioning, and subsequently on the parts only as they relate to the overall functioning of the whole system. The parts have meaning only in their relatedness to the whole. Each part is perceived as functional or dysfunctional in relation to its consequence for the larger system. The systems which are most frequently referenced as analogous to the social system are the human body and the well functioning machine. The logic of this theoretical position also dictates that the existence of a part (not unlike a heart or a liver) is itself evidence of its utility or function. An individual part does not evolve unless it is functional.[3] The parts are generated and adapted based on their functional utility for the whole. The parts facilitate the system's accomplishment of its goals.

Since the social system is perceived as a singular unit whose parts exist to fulfill the particular needs of the larger system, existing social institutions, organizations, groups and roles are by definition functional for "society." For example, the nuclear family as a unit and the roles adopted by individual family members must be functional in maintaining society, simply because the nuclear family has evolved, exists, and continues to be recreated.[4] The nuclear family and the educational systems function to recreate workers and parents in order to maintain the social system. In similar fashion, the "maternal instinct" is perceived to function as insurance for the biological recreation of the system parts.

An important feature of functionalist theory is that analysis of the parts (social groups, organizations, and individual roles) is significant only in relation to their consequences for the larger whole. For example, focus on the role of mother (the part) in family units becomes an issue when the role is perceived to be evolving in a way that is dysfunctional for the whole. A married woman's choice not to take on the role of mother or a single woman's choice to become a mother could be perceived as a threat to the larger system and, therefore, as dysfunctional. Consequently, the women themselves must be considered deviant. Just as with complex machinery or human bodies, the parts occasionally need to be fixed so that the whole is not jeopardized. So too, according to MacIntyre (1976), individuals sometimes need considerable encouragement to adopt a socially prescribed role. The process of socialization (schools, churches, youth groups, etc.) functions for the purpose of guiding individuals into socially appropriate roles.

The sick role, as elaborated by Parsons in 1951, and which the health care professions have adopted wholeheartedly, provides an excellent illustration of how the social system relates to the parts within the health care arena. Explicitly embedded in the conceptualization of the sick role is the mandate that an individual who becomes sick may "occupy" the sick role only on the condition that the sick individual (1) recognizes it as a temporary position, (2) seeks socially prescribed expertise for the purpose of becoming well, and (3) cooperates with the legitimate authorities in an attempt to become well and relinquish the sick role. In return, society grants the individual temporary relief from his or her other role obligations. Failure to meet any of these conditions, however, is indicative of socially inappropriate or deviant behavior since permanent adoption of the sick role removes individuals from other functionally necessary roles, such as worker or parent. Health care professionals refer to behavior which violates the third condition (above) as noncompliant. Yet even deviance is functional for the system as a whole. Deviant behaviors serve to elicit punitive responses from the larger system which reinforce the established norms. At the same time, deviance serves to introduce change into the system. This notion of change is similar to the concept of the biological process of mutating strains of life which gradually lead to positive, adaptive functioning.

Social change was conceptualized by the functionalists as incremental, adaptive, and primarily as the consequence of incomplete socialization (Black, 1976). The aberrant functioning of individual parts (people or groups) functions to move the system, incrementally, in the direction of progress. This naturally ameliorative process reflects the significant impact of evolutionary theory on functionalism, which renders the theory unable to accommodate rapid social change. The focus of theorizing is clearly on the maintenance of system homeostasis and equilibrium rather than on change.

Functionalism continues to be a powerful, although often unarticulated, influence in nursing theory. The centrality of concepts such as role, system, equilibrium, adaptation, and homeostasis in nursing theory attests to the comprehensive integration of functionalism.[5]

SYMBOLIC INTERACTIONISM

Symbolic interactionism and the research methods used by interactionists can best be understood in contrast to the grand social theories posited by the functionalists. Symbolic interactionism departs from functionalism in both the theoretical and moral realms. Symbolic interactionism is a response, in particular, to the notions of society as an ordered, unified, and naturally evolving whole.

Interactionists raised several significant theoretical objections to the grand theories of functionalism. First, functionalist theory was perceived as inherently normative, evaluative, and conservative (Friedrichs, 1970).

Second, it was criticized for its inability to account for (let alone to predict) rapid social change. Third, it was perceived to be a much more logical and orderly account of social life than was borne out by empirical observations (Black, 1976). Fourth, the most basic unit of analysis within the functionalist system is the role which individuals come to occupy by internalizing norms and role expectations. In the functionalist system, the acting individual could not be accounted for theoretically. This inability to access the thinking, feeling individual, and consequently the understanding of the individual only in terms of his or her role functions, became known as Parson's "black box" or the "empty vessel." In effect, these phrases specify individuals in a particularly reductive fashion. For example, individuals begin as empty vessels, ready to receive and internalize the expectations (norms) of the larger social system. Individuals are determined rather than determining. The individual could only internalize norms and expectations and was not an active participant in social processes (Black, 1976). Fifth, grand theories in general were criticized for their grounding in armchair theorizing rather than in the empirical world (Glaser & Strauss, 1967). Functionalism was a logically derived rather than an empirically derived theory.

Although the works of many sociologists, philosophers, and psychologists have influenced the intellectual development of symbolic interactionism, the names most closely associated with the Chicago School include George Herbert Mead, Robert Park, W.I. Thomas, Everett Hughes, Herbert Blumer, and Howard Becker (Fisher & Strauss, 1979). Chicago style symbolic interactionism is most comprehensively articulated in the work of Herbert Blumer (Blumer, 1969).[6]

Symbolic interactionism is theoretically focused on the acting individual rather than on the social system. For the interactionist, analysis begins with the acting individual rather than with the larger system. The direction of analysis is from the individual up through social groups, organizations, and institutions rather than from the system down through the parts to the individual role. In contrast to grand theorists who begin with the theory and then take the theory into the world in an attempt to validate it empirically, interactionists begin in the empirical world and build their theories from there.

Symbolic interactionism is a social-psychological theory of social action. The central concepts around which the theory is organized include: (1) the self, (2) the world, and (3) social action (Charon, 1979; Stryker, 1980; Meltzer, Petras, & Reynolds, 1975). For the symbolic interactionist, the self is composed of two components, the "I" and the "Me" (Mead, 1934). The Me component is conceptualized as the object of self-reflection, while the I component is the reflector. The Me is that part of the self that can be identified and talked about. It is who I am and can be described and defined to the self and to others. This Me is the object of internal conversations I have with myself, my self-image. A fundamental assumption of this theory is that each individual is comprised of multiple selves or multiple Me's. This notion is rather easy to grasp when thinking of the self as nurse colleague, as student, as mother, as sister, and as patient. Each individual incorporates multiple selves which may exist simultaneously, or consecutively, and which change over time. Who I am depends on which Me is experienced as most salient at the time. When I am sitting in a classroom the most salient Me is student, how I perceive myself as a student. When I am working as a charge nurse in the burn unit I have staffed for 12 years, the salient Me is very different. Who I am, therefore, depends on the Me that is called forth by the social context. This becomes acutely real for many of us when we find ourselves in a social situation in which two or more contexts overlap and multiple, conflicting selves emerge. While Turner (1962) refers to this as role conflict, the discomfort is clearly more than uncertainty over what role to perform. It is also a question of being, who I am, as much as doing, what actions to engage in.

For the interactionist, the self is socially constructed. The Me is constructed through ongoing social interaction which begins at birth, in which the individual person receives and interprets social cues from the environment. The individual "takes the role of the other" persons in the environment and tries to view him or herself as others do, or as he or she perceives others view him or her. The self is, therefore, fundamentally a social self. There can be no distinction between the individual and the social self since they are "twin born" (Cooley, 1964; Mead, 1934; Stryker, 1980; Meltzer, Petras & Reynolds, 1975).

A question concerning the difference between how the functionalist and the interactionist conceptualize the person should arise at this point. If the interactionist posits a self which is fundamentally social, created through the internalization of social cues, how then is this different from Parson's "black box" or "empty vessel?" The answer can be found in the second component of the self, the "I." (For a more in-depth discussion of the self see Mead, 1934.) The I is the active, interactive, dynamic, interpreting component of the self. As the Me is the object of self-reflection, the I is the reflector. The I interprets environmental cues, synthesizing them with other components of the self, relating them to the Me's. Rather than simply taking on a role by internalizing external expectations, the self is the accumulation of all previously experienced social interaction as interpreted and synthesized by the I. Therefore, the I component of the self is a source of individual agency, creativity, and unpredictability. Because the I is an interpreting process rather than an objective structure, the self is fundamentally a process. Consequently, the self is never a finished entity, but is continually evolving. The selves I am now are not the selves that I will be in the future or were in the past. While the present and future selves reflect the selves of the past, they are continually reinterpreted by the I through ongoing social interaction. The self is determining as well as determined; it acts as well as is acted upon.

This conceptualization of the self is a major departure from the functionalist notion of the socially determined self enacting or conforming to a role which has been predetermined or predefined. The functionalist sees role as primarily the consequence of complete or incomplete internalization of norms, a unidirectional process from the larger system down to the individual. The interactionist views role as the consequence of a dynamic, interactive process between the self and the social context.

THE WORLD

The second major concept for the symbolic interactionist concerns the world within which we live. What is crucial to understand is that "the world" refers to the social world, the world as interpreted or experienced, rather than to the physical world. The language used to designate this social world is the "object world" (Meltzer, Petras, & Reynolds, 1975). The language of "object world" is sometimes confusing to noninteractionists because of the tendency to think of objects as things with physical substance. For the symbolic interactionist, an object is anything that can be designated to the self or reflected on, including everything from physical objects to abstract concepts. Anxiety and professionalism are no less objects than are chairs and hats.

For the symbolic interactionist, objects have no inherent meaning. Their meaning is derived from how people act toward them. The meaning of a nurse, what a nurse is, is derived from how others act toward nurses. Others treating nurses as if they are intelligent, competent, sensitive members of a health care delivery team define the experience or meaning of being a nurse. On the other hand, if nurses are treated as if they are of marginal intelligence, have relatively unimportant skills and consequently have very little to offer, the "object" nurse has a very different meaning. In fact, the term "nurse" is a fundamentally different object in each of these scenarios. In similar fashion, a tree is a different object for a botanist, than it is for a lumberjack, a poet, or a hiker. The nature of the object (tree) is derived from its meaning. The meaning of the object is defined by how the person acts toward it. The poet, botanist, and lumberjack act differently toward the tree, which makes the tree a different object to each of them, just as the nurse is a different object depending on how others act toward him or her. Objects that are of almost universal concern to nurses include: nurse, patient, health, illness, and professionalism.

If objects are defined by the meaning they have for us and how we act toward them, then their characteristics (meanings) may vary from one individual to another, from one context to another and over time. In fact, the meaning or experience of being a nurse is not consistent from one individual to another, from one context to another and over time. Consequently, what is reality for one person is different from the reality of another person. Additionally, what is reality for one person at a given moment and in a particular context changes at a different moment or in a different context (under different conditions). This notion of multiple realities precludes the development of anything comparable to the operational definitions used by other research methods. To posit an operational definition assumes the validity of (in most cases) the re-searcher's reality (objects), his or her definition of the situation over that of the subjects. The interactionist as researcher is primarily concerned with discovering the realities of the subjects, the nature of the objects in their world, how they define and experience their world.

Objects are not static things, however. Just as the self evolves over time, so do objects. This process is referred to as an object career or trajectory. How I perceive the object "nurse" will change over time, as I experience being a nurse under different conditions.

THE OBJECT WORLD

For the symbolic interactionist, numerous objects comprise the world we live in. It is the cumulative nature of these objects that defines our social (object) world. However, each individual's object world is different than the object worlds of other individuals. This means that reality must be different for each of us. Defining an object world requires discovering what objects are salient to the individual's experience as well as under-standing the nature or meaning of the object for that person.

If reality (the object or social world) is different for each individual, one might ask, how then is it possible for individuals to understand or interact with each other? For the symbolic interactionist, the answer lies in what sociologists refer to as the socialization process, the social construction of the self. Individuals learn the meanings of objects by observing and interpreting how others act. As a child observes how others act toward women, the object "women" becomes defined. Socialization involves a process of "taking the role of the other" in an effort to view objects as others do. Consequently, the way we define objects is to a great extent received from those around us. Cultures, social classes, religions, clubs, and so forth are perceived as distinct groups because of their shared definitions or shared object worlds. This sharing leads to increased conformity in understanding and action. Such conformity allows us to accurately predict the behavior of those around us.

On the other hand, we have all experienced situations in which those around us seemed to have meaning systems very different from our own. This resulted in our inability to predict or anticipate their actions. Taking a trip to a foreign country or even visiting a different family can provide riveting examples of diverse meaning systems. Still, the ability we have to interact and work together under many conditions attests to the power of social interaction to general consensual (or at least approximate) meanings for members of the same social group.

Finally, for the symbolic interactionist, things are "real in their consequences" (Thomas, 1928). If we act toward women as if they are intellectually inferior to men, they will in turn act toward themselves as if they are intellectually inferior (social construction of the self), which will in turn create and sustain a social system in which women's opportunities and achievements are in fact inferior. In social terms, women will have consequently become inferior.

Realities that have been socially constructed become objectified (experienced as obdurate realities) and internalized by individuals. The larger social structure is thus perpetuated through the actions of individuals. Social institutions continue to exist and operate because we perceive them as real and act as if they are real. The socially constructed "reality" of women as intellectually inferior becomes an institutionalized social reality which determines the position of women in the social world. It is real in its consequences.

Social interaction is a series of processes which take place in the context of the social world and among individuals who experience those social worlds as real, and who, according to Berger and Luckman (1967), "apprehend the reality of everyday life as an ordered reality, (with) phenomena (that) are prearranged in patterns that seem to be independent of my apprehension of them and that impose themselves on the latter" (p. 21).

Social interaction, however, remains dependent on our ability to designate objects to each other, that is, to predict the action of others (recall that the meaning of an object lies in how individuals *act* toward the object). Our ability to interact effectively depends on our ability to understand the objects being designated as the designator understands them. Our accuracy in understanding these object designations in turn determines our ability to predict the actions of those in our social world. Those who do not understand or share our objects are often labeled mentally ill, that is, out of touch with (our) reality.

SOCIAL INTERACTION, THE SYMBOL AND SYMBOLIC INTERACTION

For the symbolic interactionist, symbols, which include both verbal and nonverbal gestures, also designate objects in our social world. Designating a symbol which is shared by those around us allows us to interact in a predictable or meaningful way. Here, interaction depends on access to shared symbols. Language provides us with a ready made reservoir of (approximately) shared symbols. These ready made symbols allow interaction to proceed smoothly in many situations. Since these symbols indicate to others how we will act toward the object in question, the symbol is itself an incipient act. As we receive these symbols from others (messages about how they will act), we can adjust our own actions accordingly.

Symbolic interaction, therefore, refers to the process of social interaction by which individuals are continually designating symbols to each other and to the self. In this way, our actions are built up during social interaction. According to Blumer (1969):

> Whatever the action in which he is engaged, the human individual proceeds by pointing out to himself the divergent things which have to be taken into account in the course of his action. He has to note what he wants to do and how he is to do it; . . . he has to take account of the demands, the expectations, the prohibitions, and the threats as they may arise in the situation in which he is acting (all objects). His action is built up step-by-step through a process of such self indication (self-designation). The human individual pieces together and guides his action by taking account of different things (objects) and interpreting their significance for his prospective action. (p. 81)

Included in this process is a determination about which self is the salient self (who am I now), the nature of the object world for the self (what is my social world), the nature of the object world for others (how others perceive me and a prediction of how they will act), and, consequently, a decision about how to act. So important is this determination that the process of taking-the-role-of-the-other is central to social action. Individuals are continually attempting to determine how other individuals are perceiving and interpreting their actions in order to predict the responses of others and to reconstruct their own lines of action. Even solitary action involves a process of taking-the-role-of-the-generalized other (Cooley, 1964; Blumer, 1969; Mead, 1934). While this process is going on, the individual is receiving cues from the environment which indicate how accurate his or her assessment has been and whether the selected course of action needs to be realigned or maintained. Thus, even the maintenance of "the same" course of action is an active process. Consequently, a symbolic interactionist is just as interested in how things (social organizations) stay the same as in how they change, which explains our interest in what others consider to be the mundane or usual.

Joint action, or interaction with others, is accomplished through a process of individuals attempting to take the role of the other person(s), determine the objects being designated (predict the action of others), select an action (verbal and nonverbal), and evaluate how the action is interpreted by others. These processes occur continuously and simultaneously. Consequently, social (symbolic) interaction is, according to Blumer (1969), a complex active series of social processes involving the "fitting together of lines of behavior of the separate participants" (p. 70). For this reason, it is impossible to understand the actions of any individual or group by extracting them from the social context within which they were created. Individual action, therefore, is always contextual.

While some sociologists are inclined to ask how an orderly system becomes disrupted, a symbolic interactionist is much more likely to wonder how order is possible. It is the fitting together of actions and the access to shared symbols which create social structure, organization, and order. Society is the sum total of processes engaged in by individuals who are acting as if a social structure exists, and are thereby creating that structure in all its complexity. Organizations do not exist outside of the individuals who create them. Social structure is continually recreated through individual actions.

This does not mean that an individual or group can simply redefine the social structure, since such a redefinition would require a change in the symbols (objects) of others. However, the ability of any group or individual to define the nature of any reality (the definition of the situation, the object, the symbol) for others is a direct measure of their power. In fact, most major social and political movements are simply battles over contested definitions or meanings. A current example is the battle over the definition of life. Debates over access to abortion are focused on when life begins, while debates over access to expensive medical treatment focus on when life ends.

GROUNDED THEORY RESEARCH

Grounded theory is a research method which was developed for the purpose of studying social phenomena from the perspective of symbolic interactionism (Glaser & Strauss, 1967). The method is designed primarily to generate theory from empirical data rather than to validate existing theory through theory testing (Knafl & Howard, 1984; Glaser & Strauss, 1967).[7] The term *grounded theory*, therefore, is used to designate theory and theory development which are grounded in empirical data as opposed to theory that is logically derived. It is theory that has its beginnings in the empirical world.

Grounded theory research, including methods of data collection and analysis, the generation of research and interview questions, and the relationship between the researcher and the data emerges from the theoretical framework of symbolic interactionism. Consequently, the grounded theory method departs significantly from both qualitative and quantitative methods which are rooted in other theoretical frameworks.

Role of the Researcher

Rather than attempting to remain neutral, detached, and objective, the grounded theory researcher intentionally becomes immersed in the world of the research subjects. The researcher attempts to discover what that world is like, how it is constructed and experienced (Blumer, 1969; Schatzman & Strauss, 1973; Chenitz & Swanson, 1986). Just as individuals interact with each other through a process of "taking the role of the other," so too, the grounded theory researcher attempts to take the role of the research subjects. Through this process of role-taking, the researcher is purposefully placing him or herself inside the object worlds of the research subjects. This is done for the purpose of understanding the objects (phenomena) and the object worlds from the perspective of the subjects themselves, as they understand them.

Optimally, the researcher should be able to maintain one foot in the world of the subjects and one foot outside that world, viewing actions from the perspective of the subjects while standing back and asking questions about what the subjects take for granted. Park (1950) refers to this position in and between two worlds as "marginality." Maintaining marginality facilitates the researcher's ability to view the subject's world from the inside while maintaining the distance necessary to raise analytical questions. Examples of marginality in everyday life occur in our experiences with the coming together of diverse social groups. More dramatic examples occur as a result of a mixing of cultures, that is, the foreign exchange student learning what is socially acceptable in the new culture while maintaining his or her indigenous values. Daily activities, such as joining a new group and learning the unspoken rules (shared symbols) guiding the actions of group members, offer less dramatic examples.

A marginal status allows us to see both worlds simultaneously, to make comparisons between them, discover how they are similar, and how they are different. It not only exposes us to a new and different world but, at the same time, causes us to become more sensitive to our own world. Seeing how others perform differently raises questions for us about that which we had previously taken for granted and had not been consciously aware of. This juxtaposing of worlds and the consequent heightened sensitivity allow the researcher to observe with greater acuity than would otherwise be possible. The grounded theory researcher maximizes this phenomenon through a process of constant comparative analysis.

Taking on the perspective of the subjects, adopting it as truth or reality, is commonly referred to as "going native." When this happens, the researcher loses the heightened sensitivity that comes with a marginal position. Consequently, the researcher becomes unable, or less able, to "see" objects in the world under investigation. To overcome this difficulty, the grounded theory researcher must work to maintain marginal status by continually comparing the accounts of research subjects with each other, the researcher, and the literature. Still, two problems frequently encountered by the grounded theory researcher include both the inability to enter and to step back from the world of the subjects.

Common to most beginning grounded theory researchers is an inability to enter the subject's world. This occurs when the researcher is unable to temporarily relinquish or bracket his or her perspective as the paramount reality (Schatzman & Strauss, 1973). For example, in a study of family caregivers, the researcher discovered that family caregivers had very different definitions of caregiving (the object) than the definition (another object) which was found in the literature and used by health care professionals (Bowers, 1987). The researcher, being also a health care professional, arrived at the study with an internalized definition of caregiving which matched that found in the literature but which differed from that held by the families. Families perceived caregiving as much more akin to "psychosocial care" while the researcher's definition was based on instrumental tasks such as bathing, lifting, or feeding. If the researcher had continued to use the task definition of caregiving to study what families were doing, he or she would have missed most of what the families experienced as caregiving. By accepting marginal status (which means that you, the researcher, are not expert in defining the object), the researcher is able to discover an entirely new object—in this case, caregiving as the families perceived it.

Common to researchers investigating areas in which they are also employed is an inability to step back from the world of the research subject. In this situation, the researcher is investigating an object or an object world of which he or she is already a member. For example, a graduate student, who was working as a hospital discharge planner while studying how patients perceived the discharge planning process and how well discharge planners collaborate with their patients about home care needs, had difficulty taking the role of the patient. The student continued to define home care need (object) from the perspective of the nurse (Harke, 1987). By eventually being able to bracket *her* definition of what the patients needed, she was able to see "home care needs" from the perspectives of the patients. Comparing home care needs as defined by the discharge planner (an object) to home care needs as perceived by the patients (a different object) highlighted inconsistencies between these perspectives which often lead to noncompliance.

Grounded theory analysis is conducted in groups of individuals who often have very diverse interests and areas of expertise. The combined participation of individuals who are knowledgeable about the subject, as well as those who are not, enhances the marginal position of the group.

The Research Process

Grounded theory differs from most other research methods in relation to the sequencing of steps in the research process. The phases of literature review, question/hypothesis generation, and data collection and analysis occur simultaneously rather than as a sequence of distinct phases. The ongoing process of data analysis guides the development of interview questions and sample selection. As data are collected and analyzed, the interview questions, research questions, and hypotheses change. This, in turn, leads to changes in data collected and subjects sampled (theoretical sampling).

Generating Interview Questions

Grounded theory researchers use both formal and informal interviews to collect data. Participant observation, which allows the researcher to observe, participate in, and ask questions about those observations, is ideal. Often, however, the researcher's access to the subjects is much more circumscribed, so that formal interviews must be relied on for data collection (Chenitz & Swanson, 1986; Strauss, 1987).

When using formal interviews, the grounded theory researcher generally begins the research process with a fairly general research question. For example, in the study of family caregivers the initial research question was "What is it like to care for an aging family member?" That is, what is it like to be in the object world of family caregivers? or what is the object family caregiving? A more specific research question assumes that the researcher already knows what the object is—that is, knows the definition or experience of family caregiving as the family caregiver knows it. However, this is more than the grounded theory researcher is willing to assume at this point. Taking on a specific, operational definition here often precludes the discovery of previously unknown categories. To overcome such initially proscriptive definitions, the discovery process is *central* to grounded theory research.

The researcher next invites the research subjects to explain or describe the object (family caregiving). It is crucial for the researcher not to provide the subjects with a definition of family caregiving. In a sincere attempt to be as helpful as possible, many research subjects request such a definition and try to construct their responses around the researcher's expectations. For example, if supplied with a definition of caregiving that includes "has aging relative living in the same home," a potential research subject who spends many hours each week caring for a frail parent who lives nearby might eliminate him or herself from the study altogether.

Early interview questions are also constructed in a way that gives subjects permission to define the object in the way they perceive it. Initial interview questions, therefore, must communicate the researcher's acceptance of the subject as an expert in describing the object (category) being investigated. This mandate is often difficult for both research subject and researcher. The researcher may find it difficult to bracket cherished (and hard-earned) commitments to a particular perspective while the research subject often finds it difficult to take on the role of the expert.

In the caregiving study referred to above, one of the initial interview questions was "You tell me that you have been taking care of your mother for 10 years. You must have a lot to say about what that experience is like. I'd like you to tell me what it's like to be a caregiver for an aging family member."

After such an opening question, there may be very little need for further prompting. If a subject responds with a request for clarification or more specific questions, a frequently effective approach is to emphasize the subject's position as expert. One possible response follows:

> As health care professionals we know a lot about how to treat illnesses and what we want patients and their caregivers to do. What we don't know is what it feels like to be living with those illnesses or treatment programs. When it comes to family caregiving and how it feels, the real experts are the family caregivers themselves. You're the ones who can tell us what it's like.

Other available and effective strategies include asking the subject to image how he or she would respond:

> Pretend you are attending a caregiver support group and a new member comes in. She says that her mother has just developed a chronic illness and that she will be caring for her mother. She then turns to you and asks you to tell her what it's like. What would you say?

Early Data Analysis

Discovering and describing the characteristics (dimensions) of the objects (categories) and identifying the salient objects (core categories) in the object world are the first steps in a grounded theory analysis (Chenitz & Swanson, 1986). This requires a careful line-by-line analysis (open coding) of interview transcripts, (Schatzman, in press; Chenitz & Swanson, 1986; Strauss, 1987) focusing on which categories, subcategories and dimensions the subject provides. For example, in the caregiving study, telephone contact with the first caregiver subject revealed a dimension of caregiving that the researcher had not previously considered. The subject explained to the researcher that "You can't come to my home. I don't want my mother to hear our conversation because she doesn't know that I'm taking care of her. She'd get really depressed if she knew." This woman had been taking care of her mother for 15 years. When she was questioned during the interview about her earlier comments, the caregiver described how her mother was unaware of the debilitated state she was in and was consequently unaware of her need for supervision. The caregiver subject then provided a detailed description of *hidden* caregiving, a newly discovered dimension of caregiving which was grounded in the data.

Dimensions of caregiving discovered during this first interview included: visibility (hidden or open) of caregiving; purpose of caregiving (this varied tremendously); difficulty of the work; predictability of the caregiving needs; impact of caregiving on social relationships; impact of caregiving on family relationships; impact of caregiving on caregiver-care receiver relationship; financial cost of caregiving; caregiver's perceived consequences of not providing care; and so forth.

It is not unusual for a line-by-line analysis of one interview to yield 10–20 dimensions of the category being studied. Each new dimension identified raises theoretical possibilities which direct the researcher in the development of new interview questions and the selection of research subjects. Following the analysis of each new interview, the researcher develops interview questions and selects research subjects that will provide comparisons along selected dimensions. For example, the researcher might decide to sample a caregiver whose caregiving work is not hidden. The dimensions identified from the second interview would then be compared to those identified during the first interview. This process of analysis continues until the researcher discerns *saturation* (Glaser & Strauss, 1967): that point from which the researcher cannot discover new dimensions in the data being collected.

Following each interview, a dimensional map or matrix is developed which visually displays the salient dimension(s) and the nature of their relationships to the central category and to each other. Each subsequent dimensional matrix represents not only the most recent interview but all previous interviews as well. Eventually, the researcher develops a matrix which displays the core category, the subcategories, and the related dimensions. For example, comparisons between interviews with caregivers who perceived their caregiving as hidden and those who perceived their caregiving as open revealed a consistent distinction between these two groups. Caregivers who were trying to protect their parent from knowing how ill, frail, or debilitated the parent really was and caregivers who were trying to protect the integrity of the parent-child relationship tended to try to hide their caregiving (Bowers, 1987). Those caregivers whose aim was not primarily protecting the parent in this way, did not use hidden caregiving. Thus, the visibility of caregiving (hidden or open) was determined by the purpose of caregiving (protection of personal identity and relationship).

Subsequent interviews with caregivers revealed that in each instance of protective caregiving, hidden caregiving strategies were used. Interview data are also compared along the other discovered dimensions. The processes of coding data into categories, their dimensions and subdimensions, and comparing subsequent interviews along selected dimensions (axial coding), form the foundation of grounded theory analysis (Strauss, 1987). As relationships among the categories and dimensions are discovered, tentative hypotheses are raised. The hypotheses are tested by the selection of subjects who can provide comparative cases. With each new analysis hypotheses can be confirmed, revised, or discarded (Strauss, 1987).

Identifying and sampling subjects whose accounts will provide comparisons along selected dimensions is known as theoretical sampling. Theoretical sampling is the intentional selection of subjects for the facilitation of the constant comparative analysis (Strauss, 1987). Interview questions also shift to focus on those dimensions which have been integrated into the developing theory.

The inability to predict which subjects will be sought to accomplish theoretical sampling and how interview questions evolve create some difficulties in writing and submitting research proposals. Human subjects' approval is generally contingent on the ability to give assurances about each of these processes at the proposal stage. For this reason, it is often advisable to include categories of subjects which may or may not be sampled and to submit a wide range of possible interview questions for approval by human subjects.

Eventually, the researcher will develop a dense dimensional matrix or diagram of how the categories, subcategories, dimensions, and subdimensions interrelate. At this point, it will be clear to the researcher when (under what conditions) the new grounded theory seems to be operating. For example, in the study of caregivers, the researcher would state that when the caregiver's paramount purpose is to protect the parent from illness-related knowledge that would threaten the parent's identity, the caregiver will use hidden caregiving. The caregiver's central purpose is the condition which determines the type of care provided. The researcher is then ready to make a theoretical statement about one type of caregiving (protective), and under what conditions it occurs (purpose).

Consistent with the framework of symbolic interaction, the grounded theory researcher is interested in the social processes by which "reality" is constructed or maintained. Consequently, an important theoretical category for the grounded theory researcher is the strategy(ies) used by the actors (subjects) involved. Very often the core category is itself a process (Johnson & Parrell, 1986; Bowers, 1987; Glaser, 1978; Chenitz & Swanson, 1986). This emphasis on process rather than structure is reflected in the propensity of grounded theory researchers to use gerunds (Glaser, 1978; Fagerhaugh, 1986; Strauss, 1987).

First, the researcher defines the core category (protective caregiving) and other related categories (in this case, three other types of caregiving). Next the researcher identifies the strategies used by subjects to carry out the phenomenon being studied, that is, how the actors orient their actions in relation to the object. Frequently, the researcher discovers that the actors involved have very different perceptions about the phenomenon in question and, consequently, act differently in relation to that phenomenon. In the case of the caregiving study, interviews with caregivers, elderly parents, and health care professions reveal some systematic differences in perceptions of these three groups. For example, family caregivers perceived their caregiving very differently than did professionals, and so oriented their actions differently. The discovery of these different perceptions raised questions for the grounded theory researcher about the consequences of different perceptions and the conditions under which they occur.

In addition to the core category and social processes/strategies, consequences and conditions are the two final theoretical categories which guide the grounded theorist. Questions about conditions and consequences can be addressed at many levels, depending on the nature of the particular study. While no single research project can address them all, those that occur consistently or repeatedly should be pursued.

In the caregiver study, the emerging theory about differences in perception might guide the researcher to shift the focus of subsequent interviews toward the consequences of different perceptions. A major consequence of this difference was that family caregivers often try to keep their elderly parent away from health care professionals and social service workers whose actions threaten the hidden nature of the caregiving. In other words, the analysis focuses on how the actors fit their lines of action together. As in most grounded theory studies, more than one consequence was identified during data analysis. Of course, the consequences will be different for different groups, so the researcher must always be clear about and specific for whom the consequences are operating.

Identifying the conditions under which a particular phenomenon occurs is also a central task of the grounded theory researcher. A constant comparative analysis of subjects along several dimensions will indicate the major conditions which are related to the phenomenon and in what way. For the family caregivers, the major conditions for the discovery of protective caregiving included:

1. The parent's loss of some cognitive functioning.
2. The caregiver's perception of this loss as threatening to the parent's self-esteem.
3. The caregiver's concern over the parent's emotional reaction to the loss of cognitive functioning.

Under these conditions, the caregiver is likely to engage in protective caregiving by hiding the care he or she is providing. The caregiver is taking the role of the professional (other), and anticipating his or her interventions, while also taking the role of the parent (other), and anticipating an assault to his or her self-esteem. The caregiver then fits his or her line of action (avoiding health care professionals) with the anticipated actions of both the health care professional and the parent. Under the condition that the parent is hopelessly demented or the caregiver does not perceive the illness or caregiving activities to be a threat to the parent's self-esteem, protective caregiving will not be engaged in. These hypotheses would then be tested by further data collection and analysis. The final grounded theory to emerge from the analysis would include all four theoretical categories (core categories, strategies, conditions, and consequences) and how they interrelate.

Grounded theory research can also be used to extend previously developed grounded theories or to test those grounded theories under new conditions. For example, a grounded theory study was designed to investigate how a change in one condition (moving the parent from home to nursing home) would alter the protective caregiving provided by family members. This second study focused on how families perceived and carried out caregiving within an institutional setting, testing the caregiving theory under a new condition and, thereby, expanding the theory (Bowers, in press).

Memoing

Memoing is a crucial process for the grounded theory researcher, serving several important purposes. First, memoing provides an ongoing record of theory development, a process which is otherwise difficult to reconstruct. The researcher uses theoretical memos to record important decisions about selective and theoretical sampling, shifts in the focus of interview questions, and tentative hypotheses. Initial memos often focus on identifying the dimensions of several categories discovered in the data. Subsequent memos are used to compare the relationships among categories, and to compare how relationships vary under different conditions. Memos become progressively more abstract and integrated as analysis proceeds.

Memos are also used to record lines of analysis that are not pursued. In any study, there are many possibilities which could be fruitfully pursued but are not for reasons of time, sponsorship, personal preference, access to subjects, and so forth. Conscious decisions about which lines of analysis to pursue constitute the selective sampling process (Strauss, 1987). These can form the basis of discussions about possible future studies that are indicated as well as the limitations of the study being conducted.

Memos are also used to record methodological decisions or problems. For example, the researcher uses methodological memos to record problems in gaining access to particular subjects or populations. Combined theoretical and methodological memos are used to record the possible impact of methodological decisions or problems on the emerging theory. Memos also serve as a reservoir for discovered categories, dimensions, and relationships that seem unconnected to the emerging theory. These ideas can be stored in memos for possible integration at a later time. This is especially useful when the researcher feels flooded by data (Strauss, 1987). Finally, memos are used to record theoretical and selective sampling needs, and interview questions that could be used to shift or narrow the focus of analysis.

Beginning researchers often experience the memoing process as mysterious and awkward. They find it difficult to write down unfinished, unintegrated, tentative thoughts, the stuff that early memos are made of. Most students or beginning researchers are very self-conscious about what they put in written form, feeling that written ideas must be finished work. This censoring process can seriously stifle the emerging analysis. Researchers must be encouraged to use memos freely, especially during the early stages of analysis. Reading a collection of early memos from a completed research project, often helps to free beginning researchers to use the memoing process effectively.

Memos can range from single word cues or observations to lengthy explorations about the relationships among categories, dimensions, conditions, and consequences. As the analysis proceeds, memos become more integrated, eventually approaching a polished form which can be incorporated into the final text. It is crucial that the researcher date all memos so that emergent analysis, important theoretical and methodological junctures, can be reconstructed accurately at a later time. The methods section of a grounded theory research report must include the identification of these junctures and decision points.

CONCLUSION

The grounded theory method differs significantly from the more traditional research methods in both theoretical foundation and research process. It is very difficult, if not impossible, to do grounded theory research without an in-depth understanding of this theoretical foundation. At the same time, accurately evaluating a grounded theory research report depends on the evaluator's knowledge of symbolic interaction and how it relates to the research process.

Grounded theory research cannot be distinguished from other methodologies by its chronological location in the generation of knowledge; that is, preliminary to other (quantitative) methods. The grounded theory method can be used to generate theory in an already highly researched area (family caregiving or discharge planning, for example) as well as in areas which have not been well researched.

Recently published texts (Strauss, 1987; Chenitz & Swanson, 1986) on the details of the grounded theory research process will provide researchers and reviewers guidelines with which to conduct and evaluate grounded theory studies. What has been, until recently, primarily an oral tradition is now accessible to a wider audience and, consequently, much more open to informed exploration and debate.

The relevance of grounded theory for nursing research must be discussed in terms of the *theoretical foundation*. The stated commitment of nursing research and practice to the patient, family, and society would certainly support the use of research methods which integrate the lived experience of those groups.

APPENDIX

Criteria for Reviewing Grounded Theory Research Reports*

1. *Content:* Grounded theory studies can be used for either theory generating or theory extending (sometimes both simultaneously). Theory generating studies are usually used to study an area that has not been extensively researched but may also be used where existing research does not adequately reflect the perspective of the subjects. Theory extending studies are appropriate to build on previous grounded theory studies. Grounded theory is based on the

*Developed for distribution through Midwest Nursing Research Society Section on Qualitative Research.

social psychological theory of symbolic interaction (Blumer, 1969). Social reality is based on the meanings that actors attribute to objects (meanings) in their social worlds rather than on inherent meanings.

2. *Background:* This section should provide a summary of existing research in the area, what research questions have been posed, and how the research area has been conceptualized in these studies. Many grounded theory studies include popular literature which provides insight into how the area is conceptualized by non-researchers. This is appropriate to include since grounded theory studies attempt to discover the various perspectives or meanings of the experience being studied.

3. *Clarity of Purpose:* The author should identify whether the purpose of the study is theory generating or theory extending. If the study is theory extending, reference must be made relevant to completed grounded theory studies. If the study is theory generating, the author should identify which perspectives currently dominate the literature.

4. *Sample:* The sample size may be very small, for example, five or six, or the sample size may be significantly larger, especially when a team of researchers is involved. The author must describe theoretical sampling decisions and may also describe selective sampling decisions. Selective sampling is guided by the initial purpose of the study as well as by constraints such as time, subject availability, and researcher interest. Theoretical sampling is guided by the emerging theory and is determined during data analysis. Significant theoretical sampling decisions should be identified.

5. *Instruments:* The researcher is the instrument. Data collection in grounded theory studies is not through surveys or other instruments. Structured interview schedules are inappropriate for grounded theory studies. In a grounded theory study, interview questions are redirected and become more focused in response to emerging theory. It is important for the author to discuss major shifts in the direction or focus of interviews. Examples of these changes and how they relate to the emerging theory are useful.

6. *Procedures:* How subjects were located and contacted should be included. If theoretical sampling necessitated a change in these procedures, the author should describe these changes and the reasons that prompted them. The author should state whether participant observation or an interview process was used for data collection. A

purely observational data collection method without the use of one of these interactional data collection methods is inappropriate for a grounded theory study. If participant observation is used, the author must describe what interactional (e.g., interview) techniques were used to discover the subjects' understanding of the researcher's observations. The author should describe where data collection took place, the length of time for interviews, and whether subjects were reinterviewed over time.

7. *Analysis:* The author must explain how data were analyzed. Grounded theory has evolved two very similar, overlapping methods of analysis. Both are considered grounded. The first uses the constant comparative method, coding data into categories and basic social process (Glaser & Strauss, 1967). The second uses a dimensional analysis which codes data focusing first on dimensions (categories) and dimensional matrixes (the relationships among categories), (Shatzman, in press). The difference between the methods is primarily in how early a constant comparative process is initiated.

Grounded theory studies focus on process rather than structure. Consequently, the central category of the study is often presented in the form of a gerund. Analysis often includes: (1) a central category (process); (2) *strategies* used by subjects to carry out the process(es); (3) *conditions* which influence the process, or the strategies and; (4) the *consequences* for the subjects involved.

The author should indicate whether the analysis was conducted in a group or individually. Some discussion of how the group composition facilitated the analysis (e.g., marginality) would be helpful. If the researcher conducted the analysis alone, he or she must discuss methods used to keep the analysis grounded in the data (e.g., in vivo coding, etc.).

Grounded theory is theory based on or grounded in the lived experiences of the subjects. Therefore, the use of external validity measures is not appropriate to determine the credibility of the grounded categories. Previously determined measures may be at odds with grounded categories. This reflects a difference between grounded and non-grounded research rather than a question of validity. A more appropriate measure of validity for a grounded study is the subjects' validation of in vivo codes.

Grounded theory is based on the social psychological theory of symbolic interaction which assumes that meanings are constantly evolving and do not remain static over time. The question of reliability, which assumes replicability is, therefore, not appropriate, is also of some significance. A parallel issue for a grounded theory study would be to identify the conditions under which the theory is expected to work.

In a grounded theory study, the results emerge over time, during the process of analysis. Data are being collected, and theory generated simultaneously rather than in a sequential process. An exception to this is when historical documents or diaries are the basis of analysis. When such non-interactional data are used, the limitations should be discussed.

8/9. *Results and Discussion:* These are frequently presented together. This section should be predominantly narrative and include adequate quotes from interviews to demonstrate that the theory is grounded in the data.

10. *Conclusions and Implications:* The author should identify implications for further research including theoretical questions raised but not pursued. Emphasis should be on the importance of explanation/understanding rather than prediction and control. The author may highlight any commonly held assumptions about the subjects being studied which the results of the study challenge. It is also helpful to discuss why these findings may differ from those presented in earlier studies.

11. *APA Format:* Rigid distinction between results and discussion section of the manuscript is inappropriate for grounded theory studies.

FOOTNOTES

[1] A second branch of symbolic interactionism, the Iowa School, also traces its roots to the University of Chicago during the same period of time. This second branch differs from the Chicago school in its extensive integration of the work of George Herbert Mead (Kuhn, 1964). All subsequent references to symbolic interactionism will be used to refer to the Chicago School.

[2] For a more in-depth discussion of functionalism and its intellectual roots see Black (1976), Meltzer, Petras, and Reynolds (1975), Fisher and Strauss (1978, 1979), Gouldner (1970), and Stryker (1980).

[3] This is not unlike the biological scientists' efforts to discover the functions of enzymes, receptor sites, etc., which have been identified but whose functions are unknown. Their efforts are based on the assumption

that the existence of the part is evidence for its unity. These assumptions are grounded in evolutionary theory which informs both physical and social theories.

[4]In addition to the theoretical limitations of the perspective, it is tautological and morally conservative. Change is internally suspect and differentness is construed as deviance. The theoretical position thus becomes a moral position. To be nonconforming or noncompliant is to commit a moral transgression which legitimizes the use of neutral social institutions to induce conformity.

[5]See MacIntyre (1976) for an excellent example of how functionalist theory operates in the daily practices of health care professionals.

[6]Although not explicitly stated, Blumer's work is continually in dialogue with these grand theories.

[7]Grounded theory research is not limited to theory generating purposes. The method can also be used for theory testing and extending; in particular, the testing and extending of previously generated grounded theories (Glaser & Strauss, 1967; Glaser, 1978; Strauss, 1987).

REFERENCES

Berger, P., & Luckman, T. (1967). *The social construction of reality: A treatise in the sociology of knowledge.* New York: Doubleday & Co.

Black, M. (Ed). (1976). *The social theories of Talcott Parsons.* Carbondale, IL: Southern Illinois University Press.

Blumer, H. (1969). *Symbolic interactionism: Perspective and method.* Englewood Cliffs, NJ: Prentice-Hall.

Bowers, B. (1987). Intergenerational caretaking: Adult caretakers and their aging parents. *Advances in Nursing Science, 9*(2), 20–31.

Bowers, B. (in press). Family caregiving in a nursing home. *The Gerontologist.*

Camic, C. (1987). Historical reinterpretation of early parsons. *American Sociological Review, 52*(4), 421–439.

Charlton, J., & Maines, D. (1980). The negotiated order approach to the analysis of social organization. Unpublished manuscript.

Charon, J. (1979). *Symbolic interactionism, an introduction, interpretation, and integration.* Englewood Cliffs, NJ: Prentice-Hall.

Chenitz, C., & Swanson, J. (1986). *From practice to grounded theory.* Menlo Park, CA: Addison-Wesley Publishing Co.

Cooley, C. H. (1964). *Human nature and the social order.* New York: Schocken Books.

Coser, L. (1977). *Masters of sociological thought.* New York: Harcourt Brace Jovanovich, Inc.

Fagerhaugh, S. (1986). Analyzing data for basic social processes. In C. Chenitz & J. Swanson (Eds.), *From practice to grounded theory.* Menlo Park, CA: Addison-Wesley Publishing Co.

Fisher, B., & Strauss, A. (1978). The Chicago Tradition: Thomas, Park and their successors. *Symbolic Interaction, 1.*

Fisher, B. M., & Strauss, A. L. (1979). George Herbert Mead and the Chicago tradition of sociology. *Symbolic Interaction, 2*(1), 9–26.

Friedrichs, R. (1970). *A sociology of sociology.* New York: The Free Press.

Glaser, B. (1978). *Theoretical sensitivity.* Mill Valley, CA: The Sociology Press.

Glaser, B., & Strauss, A. (1967). *The discovery of grounded theory.* New York: Aldine Publishing Company.

Gouldner, A. (1970). *The coming crisis in western sociology.* New York: Basic Books.

Harke, J. (1987). Decision making in discharge planning: Patient perspectives. Unpublished master's thesis, University of Wisconsin-Madison, School of Nursing, Madison, WI.

Knafl, K., & Howard, M. (1984). Interpreting and reporting qualitative research. *Research in Nursing and Health, 7*(1), 17–24.

Kuhn, M. (1964). Major trends in symbolic interaction theory in the past twenty-five years. *Sociological Quarterly, 5*(1), 61–84.

Johnson, M., & Parrell, S. (1986). The work of ambulatory level nurses: A grounded theory analysis of content and process. Unpublished master's thesis, University of Wisconsin-Madison, School of Nursing, Madison, WI.

MacIntyre, S. (1976). Who wants babies? The social construction of "instincts." In D. Barker & S. Allen (Eds.), *Sexual divisions and society: Process and change* (pp. 150–173). Tavistock Publications.

Mead, G. H. (1934). *Mind, self and society.* Chicago: University of Chicago Press.

Meltzer, B., Petras, J., & Reynolds, L. (1975). *Symbolic interactionism: Genesis, varieties, and criticism.* London: Routledge & Kegan Paul.

Merton, R. (1973). *The sociology of science.* Chicago: The University of Chicago Press.

Park, R. E. (1950). *Race and culture.* New York: The Free Press.

Parsons, T. (1951). Illness and the role of the physician. *American Journal of Orthopsychiatry, 21,* 452–460.

Schatzman, L. (in press). *Dimensional analysis: Conditions and grounds.*

Schatzman, L., & Strauss, A. (1973). *Field research: Strategies for a natural sociology.* Englewood Cliffs, NJ: Prentice-Hall.

Strauss, A. (1987). *Qualitative analysis.* New York: Cambridge University Press.

Strauss, A. (1978). *Negotiations, varieties, contexts, processes and social order.* San Francisco: Jossey-Bass Publishers.

Stryker, S. (1980). *Symbolic interactionism.* Menlo Park, CA: The Benjamin/Cummings Publishing Co.

Thomas, W. I. (1928). *The child in America.* New York: Alfred Knopf.

Turner, R. (1962). Role taking: Process versus conformity. In A. Rose (Ed.), *Human behavior and social processes* (pp. 20–39). Boston: Houghton-Miflen.

Futures Research

Jan L. Lee

INTRODUCTION

The future is now. The future is all around us. Today's decisions shape the future. Today's leaders must be future-oriented. We are the future.

Each of these assertions makes an implicit statement about a particular conception of the future. Each also rests on one or more implicit assumptions about the future. An individual's conception of the future constrains that individual's expectations to effect, or manage, the future. Interest in the future, and a desire to do more than just experience the future when it happens, are key motivating factors for the design and implementation of futures research.

FUTURES RESEARCH

Futures research is a means for augmenting the capabilities of persons and organizations to cope intelligently with the increasing uncertainty, rapidity of change, and complex interrelationships operant in today's world (Morrison, Renfro, & Boucher, 1984). The function of futures research is to provide decision makers with relevant information and analysis, in order to improve long-range planning.

For futures researchers, "long-range" refers to the fact that the operating conditions present during the implementation phase are expected to differ greatly from those present during the planning phase. The forecasting of such changes is an essential part of futures research.

Forecasting, Not Prediction

Futures research does not predict the future. Prediction implies certainty. Forecasting, however, encompasses probabilities, implies alternative views of the future, and thereby accounts for uncertainty.

To further clarify the difference between predictions and forecasts allow me to present an example. The statement, "One out of three American males will develop coronary artery disease by age 45, by the year 2000," is a prediction of what *will* happen. In contrast, the statement, "There is a 70 percent probability that all in-hospital patient care data will be entered at bedside terminals, by the year 1995," is a forecast of what *may* happen or what is *likely* to happen. Futures research, therefore, can be helpful in differentiating between unnecessary and unavoidable uncertainty (Helmer, 1983). Thus, forecasting is a vital component of futures research.

Purpose and Uses

The major purpose of futures research is to assist in formulating alternative futures. In so doing, futures research enhances understanding of what is changing (trends), what may happen (forecasts), and what ought to be done (policy proposals or specific prescriptions for action) (Marien, 1987).

Becoming aware of alternative futures, through futures research, also can be enabling. Depending on such factors as philosophy and temperament, futures research can be used to improve individual response to the uncertainty of the future. Alternatively, futures research can be used to help take responsibility for shaping the future. Futures researchers (Harman & Schwartz, 1978) have termed the first stance "anticipatory response planning" and the second "intervention assessment" (p.791). Furthermore, anticipatory response planning is characterized by a reactive posture, while intervention assessment illustrates a more proactive posture.

Applications to Nursing.   Futures research methods have been utilized by nurse researchers, with one particular method, the Delphi technique. An early Delphi was conducted by Lindeman (1975) for the purpose of determining priorities for clinical research in nursing. A more recent Delphi, conducted by Henry et al. (1985), sought to specify and prioritize significant researchable problems in nursing administration.

Still another Delphi, conducted by the Nursing 2020 Study Group, explored the future of hospital-based nursing in the years 2000 and

2020 (Warnick & Sullivan, 1988). Other Delphi studies reported by nurses have addressed diverse topics, including curriculum planning (Sullivan & Brye, 1983); exploration of health care, nursing practice, education, and administration in 1992 (Hill, 1984); and identification of patient behavioral indicators of acceptance of nurse practitioners (Facione & Facione, 1985).

HISTORY

Futures research, in various forms, has been a part of humankind ever since time-orientation (i.e., a sense of time-past, time-present, and time-future) was first perceived. The ancient Greeks handed down their version of futures research via the story of the gods receiving the oracle at Delphi. In the judeo-christian tradition, the Bible also includes several books devoted to the prophets and their foretellings.

The origins of contemporary, organized futurist activity (somewhat ironically) are linked to military studies of future warfare capabilities, begun during World War II (Dickson, 1977). The first of the future-oriented "think tanks," the RAND Corporation, was established as an outgrowth of that initial military study (Helmer, 1983).

During the 1960s, two independent organizations devoted to futures research were founded: the World Future Society, in 1966, and the Institute for the Future, in 1968. The World Future Society, an association for the study of alternative futures, is a non-profit educational and scientific organization, which acts as an impartial clearinghouse for a variety of differing perspectives. The Society does not take positions on what will—or what ought to—happen in the future (Marien, 1987). The Institute, on the other hand, espouses a more normative approach, encompassing both the decisions to be made (what ought to happen) and subsequent policy implications (how to make it happen) (Helmer, 1983).

By 1970, the futures research process was mandated by Congress via the National Environmental Protection Act, which required that an environmental study be conducted prior to instituting major technological innovations with the potential to harm the environment. Further governmental actions, principally through the establishment of the Office of Technology and Assessment and the "foresight" provision required for all newly-proposed legislation, have illustrated the importance of identifying possible consequences of future, alternative actions (Harman & Schwartz, 1978).

The futures movement also has had its popular side, which was born with Alvin Toffler's (1971) *Future Shock*. This movement crested in the early 1980s, accompanied by such futures classics as *The Aquarian Conspiracy* (Ferguson, 1980), *The Third Wave* (Toffler, 1981), and *Megatrends* (Naisbitt, 1983).

By 1987, however, some retrenchment in futures activities was noted. The Center for Futures Research at the University of Southern California closed its doors in 1987. The broad base of support provided by the business community, which had contributed to the prosperous Center during its 14-year existence, was dwindling badly, as corporations turned

Table 1
Future-related Vocabulary

Discontinuity:	A radical shift in direction or trend (such as when we have been told that Type A behavior is a cardiac risk factor and then we learn that new research indicates that Type A behavior may prolong survival by keeping persons on a health care regimen).
Econometrics:	Equations or models which describe the working of an economy (such as those which help explain health care financing in the 1980s).
Futurizing:	The process by which an outlook or institution is reoriented toward the future (such as *Nursing Outlook* becoming the official journal of the American Academy of Nursing).
Pluralistic society:	One in which a variety of groups are able to maintain both identity and some degree of autonomy (such heterogeneity has enormous implications for service providers, such as nurses).
Post-affluence:	The period of lowered living standards which many believe is now at hand (this period is also marked by increased consumerism, even in health care behaviors).
Pro-act:	To respond in advance, the opposite of react (such strategies are important as futures researchers and policy makers try to influence the future).
Wild card:	The term used to describe a major, unforeseen development that could wipe out less dramatic scenarios and projections (such as the impact on health care financing, if the Health Care Financing Administration were to be disbanded).

Adopted from Dickson (1977), pp. 241–246.

Table 2
General Futures Research Periodicals

Futures: The Journal of Planning and Forecasting

Technological Forecasting and Social Change

Futurics: A Quarterly Journal of Futures Research

Cultural Futures Research

Future Survey/FS Annual

World Futures

Impact Assessment Bulletin

Journal of Forecasting

Futures Research Quarterly

International Journal of Forecasting

Project Appraisal

Adopted from Marien (1987), p. 187.

their sights from the long-range to the short-term. Another clue to this downturn in futurism was the declaration by the *Future Survey Annual 1986* that 31 futures-related periodicals had ceased operation. Of some concern is the observation that most of these now-defunct periodicals were broadly interdisciplinary in focus. Unfortunately, this trend is gain-

Table 3
Futures-Relevant Periodicals in Health and Human Services

Milbank Memorial Fund Quarterly: Health and Society

Inquiry: The Journal of Health Organization, Provision and Financing

Aging and Work

Family Planning Perspectives

The Hastings Center Report

Journal of Health Policy, Politics, and Law

Child Abuse and Neglect

Holistic Health Review

Augustus: A Journal of Progressive Human Services

Health Policy and Education

Health Care for Women International

Journal of Public Health Policy

Health and Medicine

Health Policy Quarterly

Health Promotion

Adopted from Marien (1987), p. 191.

ing even greater momentum. Corporate mentality, which encourages a reductionist-specialist approach to futures research, is gaining in prestige while its opposite, which encourages a humanistic, holistic, and generalist approach has not been as fortunate.

Even though the pendulum appears to be swinging away from the frenetic pace and style of futures activity which marked the early 1980s, certain tangible perspectives appear to have weathered the storm. These perspectives are most obvious in vocabulary and in periodicals. See Table 1 for definitions of selected terms that arose in futures research and have now become accepted. Health care and nursing-related implications of these terms are also noted.

Numerous futures-relevant periodicals now vie for market share. Representative periodicals, focused on general futures research, are found in Table 2, while Table 3 lists selected periodicals from the field of health and human services.

PHILOSOPHY

The underlying philosophy of futures research is predicated on the fact that there are numerous alternative futures, coupled with the obligation of responsible citizens to make appropriate decisions that will impact the probabilities of those alternative futures.

This philosophy, stated in the Institute for the Future's first prospectus, was reproduced by Helmer (1983):

> There is no single, inevitable, predestined future to be predicted and prepared for; instead there are countless possible futures—some desirable, toward realization of which we may choose to devote present energies, and some undesirable, which we may work to avoid. Illuminating the range of possible future alternatives, identifying the linkages from them to present decisions, and assisting in the formulation of appropriate policies—all these are essential . . . (p. 113)

RESEARCHER CHARACTERISTICS

Persons wishing to undertake futures research would be well-advised to have a firm foundation in both qualitative and quantitative methodologies. Comfort with uncertainty, tolerance for ambiguity, and the ability to engage in lateral thinking are all important qualifications. Just as useful, though, are familiarity with statistical procedures and experience in interpreting simple and complex statistical results.

Table 4
Art Versus Science of Futures Research

Art	*Science*
Scanning	Content Analysis
Informed Opinion	Delphi Survey Nominal Group Technique QUEST Process
Lateral Thinking	Linear Projections Trend Extrapolations
Imaging	Trend-impact Analysis Cross-impact Analysis
Scenarios	Mathematical Models Computer Simulations

Adopted from Lee (1988).

The futures researcher, in an optimal sense, would maintain a holistic perspective resulting from a synergistic combination of qualitative and quantitative approaches. In reality, an investigator who undertakes futures research is most likely an established researcher is his or her own field. Again, in most cases, a researcher becomes interested in futures research methods for the purpose of addressing a problem in that specific discipline. For both of these reasons—comfort with particular methodologies and bias inherent in vested interest—one consultant, at minimum, or, preferably, an interdisciplinary group, should be involved in any futures research project. For a discussion of the potential problems inherent in such a group research approach see the section on "Implementation Challenges."

RESEARCH PROCESS

Art Versus Science

Futures research possesses elements of both art and science (see Table 4). The art of futures research employs scanning, informed opinion, lateral thinking, imaging, and scenario building. Each of these elements corresponds to more objectifiable, quantifiable, scientific techniques. Thus, scanning may be quantified via content analysis; informed opinion may be investigated via the Delphi survey, the Nominal Group Technique, or the QUEST process; lateral thinking may be compared to its more linear products, such as linear projections or trend extrapolations; imaging can be reduced to matrix manipulation via trend-impact analysis and cross-impact analysis; and scenario building can be imitated by mathematical models and computer simulations.

Representative Techniques

The art of futures research, utilizing such approaches as scanning, informed opinion, lateral thinking, imaging, and scenario building, requires information, time, and open-mindedness on the part of the investigator. Whereas scanning of multitudes of print media and formulating informed opinion in individual areas of expertise are common practices for today's information specialists (no matter the discipline), lateral thinking and imaging may present other problems for the specialist. However, specific sensitization and intensive group work may help free the specialist from the bonds of linear, reductionistic thinking.

Scenario Building.   The most concrete of the "art" techniques, scenario building, is the process of constructing histories of the future. Scenarios are descriptions of plausible alternative futures of the macroenvironment. Their principal purpose is to bound the range of uncertainty in the factors most critical to a particular decision or forecast. Scenarios serve as a collection of insights for evaluating, adjusting, and ultimately making sense out of the results of more formal methods. The process of developing scenarios is nearly as important as the resulting scenarios. The key point is: scenarios don't reduce uncertainty, they clarify it (Mandel, 1983).

Examples of scenarios found in nursing and health care literature are the description of a nurse pioneer in space (Warnick & Sullivan, 1988), the concept of a nurse engineer, linking nursing theory and nursing practice (Harrell, 1986), and a detailed accounting of future health science personnel, such as health academicians and health technical experts (Lesse, 1981).

Quantifiable "science" techniques will now be discussed. Representative techniques include the Delphi survey, the Nominal Group Technique, the QUEST process, trend-impact analysis, cross-impact analysis, and INTERAX, a computer simulation.

Delphi Survey.   The Delphi survey is one method for quantifying informed opinion. Linstone and Turoff (1975) have defined the Delphi technique as "a method for structuring a group communication process so that the process is effective in allowing a group of individuals, as a whole, to deal with a complex problem" (p. 3).

The Delphi technique replaces face-to-face debate with serial rounds of data collection conducted by an intermediary. Thus, anonymity of opinion is achieved and certain psychological factors, such as undue influence by one or more dominant personalities or the bandwagon effect, are avoided or reduced. Delphi panelists are provided with feedback on the opinions of the other panelists, usually in the form of frequency statistics. But, again, the intermediary prepares this information in a confidential manner and authorship of any particular opinion is not revealed.

Nominal Group Technique. The Nominal Group Technique (NGT) is very similar to the Delphi survey in that the NGT seeks to quantify informed opinion. The major difference is that NGT panelists meet together face-to-face to gather expert opinion (Delbecq, Van de Ven, & Gustafson, 1975). The NGT has one advantage over the Delphi survey; NGT panelists have the opportunity to expand upon their responses and to clarify any misunderstandings or misinterpretations among themselves. The disadvantage of the NGT is that psychological factors inherent in group interaction (i.e., undue influence or the bandwagon effect, mentioned above) may affect the outcome of the process.

QUEST Process. QUEST stands for Quick Environmental Scanning Technique. It is composed of four activities: (1) preparation, (2) divergent planning session, (3) scenario development, and (4) strategic options identification.

The QUEST process is designed to permit executives and planners in an organization to share their views about trends and events in future external environments that have critical implications for the organization's strategies and policies. It is a systematic, intensive, and relatively inexpensive way to develop a shared understanding of high priority issues and to focus management's attention quickly on strategic areas for which more detailed planning and analysis would be beneficial (Nanus, 1983).

Trend-Impact Analysis. This technique employs elements of probabilistic forecasting, extrapolated trends, and hypothesized external events. Trend-impact analysis could be used to investigate the following question of interest to nursing: How would the continuing increase in ambulatory, community, and home care be impacted by an external event such as preferential reimbursement patterns for *non-acute* care?

Cross-Impact Analysis. Termed by Helmer (1983) as the most promising advance beyond Delphi, cross-impact analysis is concerned with mutual interactions among future trends and events. Event-to-event and trend-to-trend impacts can be considered simultaneously (Morrison, Renfro, & Boucher, 1984).

A matrix crossing the macroenvironment and the microenvironment illustrates this point. In nursing, the microenvironment may be conceptualized in terms of practice, education/research, ethics, and finance/management. The macroenvironment may be divided into STEEP categories: Social, Technological, Environmental, Economic, and Political. A cross-impact analysis would involve identifying possible occurrences for each box (see Figure 1).

INTERAX. INTERAX, a computer-based procedure developed at the University of Southern California's Center for Futures Research, conducts cross-impact analysis via computer simulations. INTERAX brings

---

Figure 1
Illustration of a Cross-Impact Analysis Matrix
for the Macroenvironment and Microenvironment of Nursing

	S*	T*	E*	E*	P*
Practice					
Education/Research					
Ethics					
Finance/Management					

*STEEP = Social, Technological, Environmental, Economic, and Political.

together both forecasting models and human policy analysts in a strategic gaming environment (Nanus, 1983).

VALIDITY, RELIABILITY, AND GENERALIZABILITY

Probabilistic pronouncements, informed opinion, and pseudo-experimentation do not automatically yield much confidence in terms of validity and reliability criteria, to say nothing of generalizability. Each of these criteria, validity, reliability, and generalizability, can be addressed, however, within the context of futures research.

Validity of futures research can only be truly assessed by the degree to which it corresponds to the actual future. Longitudinal designs or periodic comparisons of futures research conclusions with actual occurrence would be necessary to evaluate validity.

Reliability of futures research results have varied. Rather than concentrating on reliability of results, Helmer (1983) suggests that evaluating the reliability of the problem formulation may be useful. This suggestion could be expanded to include reliability testing not only of problem statements, but also of assumptions, trends, and hypothesized surprise events.

Generalizability, as a criterion, is relevant only to the degree that the results of a futures research study spur the imaginations and clarify the intentions of policy makers. True generalizability is probably both undesirable and inadvisable; since, indeed, a major purpose of futures research is to develop and test alternative visions of the future.

Even so, validity, reliability, and, to a lesser degree, generalizability, can be enhanced by careful planning and implementation by the futures researcher. Specific variables which can improve validity, reliability, and generalizability include: (1) representativeness of the expert panel, (2) informedness of assumptions, (3) commitment of experts to the process, and (4) precision with which the study protocol is conducted.

IMPLEMENTATION CHALLENGES

Securing Funding

The first challenge for the futures researcher is to secure funding to support the project. As noted earlier, available funds for futures studies have declined as organizations have moved from long-range strategic planning to short-term management. Since futures research may be conducted using a variety of techniques, some of which are clearly less expensive to employ than others, and, since the goal of futures research is to develop alternative futures, provocative results may be obtained without huge dollar investments. Seed monies, both intramural and extramural, may be an ideal avenue to explore. After all, if a futures research project, funded by seed money, impacts policy implementation or long-range strategic planning efforts, the objectives of both the funder and the investigator will have been met.

Selecting Method and Panel

The selection of which particular futures research method or methods to use and the selection of expert panelists (if indicated by the method chosen) are vitally important decisions. Such decisions should be predicated on familiarity with method, availability of additional, consultative expertise, and the ever-present constraints of time and money. Remember, as noted earlier, selection of expert panelists should hinge on representativeness, not number.

Drowning in Data

Specific futures research methods are especially prone to this "data dump" syndrome. The methods for quantifying informed opinion (Delphi, NGT, and QUEST) are particularly prone to this problem. Clear, precise objectives and attention to study protocol will help to decrease data overload. Purposeful design decisions can be a very effective preventive strategy. For example, in the Nursing 2020 study (Warnick & Sullivan, 1988), the study group made a conscious decision not to solicit panelist written comments until round three of the Delphi survey. Thus, only panelists' numeric forecasts and sufficiency-of-information scale responses were collected in round two; round three data included these responses plus written comments.

Staying Data-Based

Since futures researchers often have a vested interest in the projects they undertake, there is a very real danger of introducing bias into the research process, especially at the stages of data interpretation, conclusion formulation, and recommendation proposal.

A helpful suggestion for trying to decrease bias is for the researcher or research group to repeatedly ask the following questions:

1. Is this what the data are actually showing?
2. Am I (are we) reading something into the data?
3. Is this conclusion/recommendation justified *on the basis of the data?*
4. What other conclusions/recommendations *emerge from the data?*

Surviving Group Research

Group research, or research by committee, has advantages and disadvantages. Positively, a group research effort has the potential benefits of multiple persons' expertise, insight, contacts, and work time. Negatively, a group research effort has the potential risks of unclear or competing objectives, unclear or competing leadership, ill-defined group member roles and expectations, hidden agendas, and conflicting loyalties. Long-recognized issues of collaborative research, such as distribution of workload versus authorship credit, should be addressed early on in the process.

Without a doubt, the best approach to decreasing the problems of group research is to heed the voice of experience, whether a colleague's or your own. Group research can be creative and invigorating, or frustrating and ineffective. It really depends on the players, the rules, and how they play the game.

THEORY DEVELOPMENT

Possible uses of futures research methods in theory development for nursing could include identifying research priorities within specific nursing theories, achieving consensus from nurse experts regarding theory components within and between specific nursing theories, and simulating the consequences of different theoretical assumptions upon resulting theoretical propositions and other theory formulations, both within and between nursing theories.

Any such futures research project must not end with the study results themselves. The "next step," equally important as the original study, is to implement and test the study conclusions and recommendations.

CONCLUSION

Futures research methods provide a mechanism for investigators to develop alternate visions of the future. Numerous techniques have been developed to assist the researcher who desires to forecast the future. Both the art and the science of futures research are valued approaches. Replete with challenges and opportunities, futures research is an important adjunct to the strategic planning process.

REFERENCES

Delbecq, A. L., Van de Ven, A. H., & Gustafson, D. H. (1975). *Group techniques for program planning: A guide to nominal group and Delphi processes.* Glenview, IL: Scott, Foresman.

Dickson, P. (1977). *The future file.* New York: Avon.

Facione, N. W., & Facione, P. A. (1985). Acceptance of nurse practitioners: Patient behavioral indicators. *Nurse Practitioner. 10*(1), 55–57.

Ferguson, M. (1980). *The aquarian conspiracy: Personal and social transformation in the 1980s.* Los Angeles: J. P. Tarcher.

Ferkiss, V. C. (1977). *Futurology: Promise, performance, prospects.* The Washington Papers, Vol. 5, no. 50. Beverly Hills: Sage Publications.

Harman, W. W., & Schwartz, P. (1978). Changes and challenges of futures research. In J. Fowles (Ed.), *Handbook of futures research* (pp. 791–801). Westport, CT: Greenwood Press.

Harrell, J. (1986). Needed: Nurse engineers to link theory and practice. *Nursing Outlook, 34*(4), 196–198.

Helmer, O. (1973). *The use of expert opinion in international-relations forecasting.* Los Angeles: University of Southern California Center for Futures Research, #M7.

Helmer, O. (1983). *Looking forward: A guide to futures research.* Beverly Hills: Sage Publications.

Henry, B., Moody, L.E., O'Donnell, J., Pendergast, J., & Hutchinson, S. (1985, October). *National nursing administration research priorities study.* Report to Division of Nursing. Washington, DC: United States Public Health Service.

Hill, B. A. S. (1984). A Delphi application health care, practice, education, and education administration; circa 1992. *Image: The Journal of Nursing Scholarship, 16*(1), 6–8.

Lee, J. L. (1988). Appendix B: Overview of futures research. In M. Warnick & T. Sullivan (Eds.), *Nursing 2020: A study of the future of hospital-based nursing* (pp. 53–58). New York: National League for Nursing.

Lesse, S. (1981). *The future of the health sciences: Anticipating tomorrow.* New York: Irvington.

Lindeman, C. A. (1975). Delphi survey of priorities in clinical nursing research. *Nursing Research, 24*(6), 434–441.

Linstone, H. A., & Turoff, M. (Eds.). (1975). *The Delphi method: Techniques and applications.* Reading, MA: Addison-Wesley.

Mandel, T. F. (1983). Futures scenarios and their uses in corporate strategy. In K. J. Albert (Ed.), *The strategic management handbook* (pp. 10–21). New York: McGraw-Hill.

Marien, M. (Ed.). (1987). *Future survey annual 1986*. Bethesda, MD: World Future Society.

Morrison, J. L., Renfro, W. L., & Boucher, W. I. (1984) *Futures research and the strategic planning process: Implications for higher education*. ASHE-ERIC Higher Education Research Report No. 9. Washington, DC: Association for the Study of Higher Education.

Naisbitt, J. (1982). *Megatrends: Ten new directions transforming our lives*. New York: Warner Books.

Nanus, B. (1983). *Futures research and policy research*. Los Angeles: University of Southern California Center for Futures Research, #M42.

Nanus, B. (1982). QUEST—quick environmental scanning technique. *Long Range Planning, 15*(2), 39–45.

Sullivan, E., & Brye, C. (1983). Nursing's future: Use of the Delphi technique for curriculum planning. *Journal of Nursing Education, 22*(5), 187–189.

Toffler, A. (1971). *Future shock*. New York: Bantam.

Toffler, A. (1981). *The third wave*. New York: Bantam.

Warnick, M., & Sullivan, T. (Eds.). (1988). *Nursing 2020: A study of the future of hospital-based nursing*. New York: National League for Nursing.

Meta-Analysis

Mary Colette Smith

Today there is a growing proliferation of information and vehicles for dissemination within nursing. To remain conscientious of these data, the methods used to analyze them, and the rectitude of conclusions drawn from them, a dramatic change in the way we identify, access, retrieve, and store printed materials for use is necessary. More importantly, there is a need for contemporary research reviewing to be more systematic than the traditional narrative (Glass, McGaw, & Smith, 1981; Wolf, 1986).

As a mode of inquiry, meta-analysis is the application of the research process to a collection of studies (Smith & Naftel, 1984). In meta-analysis, results of multiple and diverse investigations are transformed into a common metric, yielding a more comprehensible body of literature on a given topic. With this technique, contradictory findings of primary research reports are often found not to be conflicting, but rather to be opposite ends of a distribution of related results (Kulik, Kulik, & Cohen, 1979).

The systematic combining of single study results, according to the rigors of meta-analytic synthesis strategies, provides a link between multiple primary research results and their integration into the discipline (Cooper, 1984). It also helps organize a body of literature and facilitates understanding of available information on a topic (Friedman & Booth-Kewley, 1987). Quantitatively, meta-analysis yields effect magnitudes, variability explanations, interrelationships, and differences. Qualitatively, meta-analysis yields arrays and lists of descriptive data amenable to identification of patterns. From either approach, hypotheses can be generated for new primary studies or additional meta-analyses. Updates of literature can be added to the existing corpus of studies on a regular

77

basis to keep state-of-the-art literature on the phenomenon current.

Meta-analytic techniques tease out conditions and situations under which circumstances occur, providing insights into phenomena otherwise unobtainable. A meta-analysis of three decades of research, on "type A and type B behaviors," for example, revealed that the image of the workaholic, hurried, impatient individual is a questionable indicator of coronary proneness. Instead, negative emotions such as depression, aggressive competition, anger, and anxiety emerged as personality characteristics associated with coronary heart disease (Booth-Kewley & Friedman, 1987).

Applying research processes used in single studies to a group of studies requires a high level of conceptualization regarding the nature of nursing, the phenomenon under investigation, primary research processes and methodologies, and meta-analysis. Just as the task demands, and as cognitive operations of composing and summarizing are fundamentally different from one another (Hidi & Anderson, 1986), so are the tasks and operations required in meta-analysis compared with those of primary research. A distinctly scholarly approach is required to make decisions regarding technical treatment of the primary research data. As any professional person must be able to evaluate a single research report for merit, likewise, consumers of meta-analysis must be sufficiently informed to assess research synthesis processes and products.

The purpose of this chapter is to provide an overview of meta-analysis. A general background of meta-analysis, conceptual issues, design and procedural aspects, concerns, evaluation criteria, and the future of meta-analysis in nursing are presented.

BACKGROUND

The term "meta-analysis" was coined by Gene Glass in 1976. The underlying processes of combining results from many studies, however, had been available since the 1930s. Related to agricultural research (Hedges & Olkin, 1985; Wolf, 1986), the need then was to assess a combined effect across situations of different climatic conditions, soil variations, and crops. Early statisticians who attempted to combine evidence across studies included Tippet (1931), Fisher (1932), Pearson (1933), and Cochran (1937).

More recently, works by Glass, McGaw, and Smith (1981), Cooper (1982), Hedges and Olkin (1985), Hunter, Schmidt, and Jackson (1982), Jackson (1980), Light and Pillemer (1984), Orwin and Cordray (1985), Rosenthal (1984), Stock et al. (1982), and Wolf (1986) have served as models and sources of meta-analyses in a variety of disciplines. Although the common denominator of "research synthesis" is present in all these studies, readers should recognize that there are different approaches to meta-analytic methods. Distinctions among these and suggestions for their use are easily identifiable in the literature (Bangert-Drowns, 1986).

A recent computer search for meta-analysis articles over an 18-month period yielded 340 titles from multiple disciplines. Some topical examples of meta-analyses include: exercise and sport (Thomas & French, 1986); alcohol consumption (Hull & Bond, 1986); psychological treatment of coronary prone behavior (Nunes, Frank, & Kornfeld, 1986); marital status and subjective well-being (Haring-Hidore et al, 1985); effects of electroconvulsive therapy (Janicak et al, 1985); paternal absence and sex role development (Stevenson, 1985); psychological predictors of heart disease (Booth-Kewley & Friedman, 1987); full moon effects (Rotton & Kelly, 1985); food and nutrition related research (Axelson, Federline, & Brinberg, 1985); patient education (Mullen, Green, & Persinger, 1985; Posovac, 1980); psychological intervention effects on recovery from surgery and heart attack (Mumford, Schlesinger, & Glass, 1982); medical versus surgical treatment of coronary artery disease (Lynn & Donovan, 1980); deinstitutionalization in mental health (Straw, 1983); family studies (Wampler, 1982); only child literature (Falbo & Polit, 1985); childbirth education (Jones, 1983); psychoeducational interventions (Devine & Cook, 1983); maternal–infant interaction (Turley, 1985; Vance, 1986); and nonnutritive sucking in premature infants (Schwartz, Moody, Yarandi, & Anderson, 1987). Louis, Fineberg, and Mosteller (1985) summarized several meta-analysis findings in public health as the basis for hypothesis generation. Sacks, Berrier, Reitman, Ancona-Berk, and Chalmers (1987) presented an analysis of 86 meta-analyses on randomized controlled trials from 51 medical journals. Special issues of *Clinical Psychology Review* (Michelson, 1985), the *Journal of Nutritional Education* (Johnson & Johnson, 1985), the *Journal of Consulting and Clinical Psychology* (Garfield, 1983), and *Statistics in Medicine* (Colton, Freedman, & Johnson, 1987) have been devoted to meta-analysis.

The appearance of meta-analysis in such a wide range of fields of study suggests increasing recognition of the need for development of meta-analytic strategies to integrate quantification, computer technology, scholarship, and information into a comprehensible unity for consumers.

EPISTEMOLOGICAL ISSUES

In meta-analysis, as in any research endeavor, there are epistemological issues concerning the nature of knowledge, science, theory, research, measurement, and the phenomenon under study (Smith, 1987, 1988). Table 1 depicts epistemological issues underlying modes of inquiry in general, and the assumptions made by researchers using meta-analysis in particular. The general epistemological framework structuring meta-analysis is viewed by researchers as *a zone of knowledge conceived as a universe of elements and their properties, derived from an explicit formal object of the discipline, to yield tentative formulations reducing uncertainty regarding the phenomenon under study.*

The search for a unified body of knowledge is the underlying epistemological motivation of researchers using meta-analysis. An obvious question follows: Can such a unified whole exist in scientific knowledge or must we accept the inevitability of fragmentation of information? Researchers using meta-analysis implicitly assume the contrary, and that fragmentation can be overcome.

The selection of concepts for meta-analysis also raises questions of appropriate standards and what studies should be included and

Table 1
Epistemological Issues in Meta-Analysis

Inquiry
* Search for a unified whole (Dewey, 1938)

Knowledge
* Question of standards (Harré, 1972)
* Selection of concepts (Harré, 1972)
* Zones for inclusion and exclusion (Maritain, 1959)

Science
* Problems of classification (Mukherjee, 1983)
* Formal object of the discipline (Dagenais, 1972; Maritain, 1959)
* Conceived universe (Rudner, 1966)

Theory
* As core for knowledge extension (Munevar, 1981)
* Central to use of experimental design (Blalock, 1982; Suppe, 1974)
* Hazards of crossing disciplines with constructs (Whitley, 1983)
* Generation of formulations (Rudner, 1966)

Research
* Data sets arise from particular contexts (Mukherjee, 1983)
* Nonmeasurability and noncomparability of phenomena (Blalock, 1984)
* Situation specificity of research (Blalock, 1984)
* Complexity of phenomena (Black, 1954)

Meta-Analysis
* Insight beyond a single case (Lonergan, 1980)
* Commonalities from aggregates as the basis for fundamental knowledge (Shapiro, 1984)
* Greater confidence from aggregates than single study results (Hendrick & Jones, 1972)

excluded. This, in turn, raises deeper issues of classification of concepts and the formal object and conceived universe of the discipline. The central importance of theory as the core for knowledge extension must always be kept in sight. In the selection of studies, researchers face a further hazard: of crossing disciplines concerned with constructs of the same name. However, researchers must also recognize that the formulation and measurement of the same construct and concept may differ significantly from one discipline to another.

Even within a single discipline, the problem of the situational specificity of research remains. Data sets arise from particular contexts, and many theoreticians maintain that complex phenomena measured in one situation are not comparable in a different setting. This may be particularly true in human settings. Yet researchers using meta-analysis know that insights gained from aggregates of studies provide a stronger foundation for knowledge than the results of single studies.

In addition to these considerations, one must take into account a variety of issues related to the methods and techniques of meta-analysis (Smith, 1988). Assumptions and limitations of the primary research plus those of the meta-analysis are reflected in the meta-analytic project. The results, then, are as credible as the weakest link in the chain of reasoning and substance of the meta-analysis.

DESIGN AND PROCEDURAL ASPECTS

In many respects, meta-analysis involves a traditional research methodology, specifically in regard to the elements of the process: a unit of study, a data set, and independent and dependent variables. Differences, however, do exist in the content of the elements, as illustrated in Table 2. Instead of a sample of individual subjects, the usual unit of research focus (or data set) is a group of studies. The findings and study charac-

Table 2
Design Aspects of a Meta-Analysis

Units of research endeavor:	Individual study
Data set:	Findings and study characteristics
Independent variables:	Methodological characteristics (Research related)
	Substantive characteristics (Phenomenon related)
Dependent variable:	Effect

teristics, as properties of the study, constitute the data set. Researchers view the study characteristics as factors potentially contributing to the dependent variable of overall effect.

Table 3
Design Overview of a Meta-Analysis: Nursing Intervention Research

Problems:

1. What is the combined corrected relative effect size derived from nursing intervention research?
2. How much of the variability of corrected relative effect sizes can be accounted for by study characteristics?
3. Which study characteristics do and do not contribute to the combined corrected relative effect size?
4. Are the study characteristics interrelated?
5. Are there differences in effect sizes by study characteristics comparisons?

Theoretical Bases:

Knowledge, Science, Theory, Research, Meta-Analysis, Nursing—as a transcending perspective regarding a reduction in uncertainty concerning authoritative knowledge about nursing intervention research over a designated period of time

Major Terms:

Meta-Analysis—Quantitative synthesis of nursing research through application of meta-analytic models as described by Hedges and Olkin (1985)

Nursing interventions—Identifiable action(s) by a nurse directed toward an investigator designated patient outcome

Research—Retrievable experimental studies printed in the United States from 1900 to 1983 in book, report, dissertation, or journal form

Combined corrected relative effect size—Simultaneous strength of effect expressed in Fisher's Chi-square (1932) and z values based on k independent tests of significance

Study characteristics—Methodological variables include: publication date, form, source derivation, number of authors, funding, type of experimental design, sampling method, sample size, and quality of study. Substantive variables include: client and nurse age, gender, sociocultural status, socioeconomic status, educational level; client diagnosis; nursing theory, non-nursing theory, concept; nursing intervention type, category, unit of service, duration; use of media, equipment; health, health deviation requisite; outcome type, category and reactivity

Design:

Descriptive, meta-analysis

Analysis:

Descriptive profile of the study characteristics revealed by the corpus of studies
Computation of corrected relative effect sizes
Regression equations, *t*-tests, and analyses of variance

Table 3 presents a design overview for the meta-analysis of a nursing intervention research project (Smith, 1988). The "bare bones" format illustrates the application of the research process from single to multiple studies through use of basic scientific research elements.

Table 4, which lists the procedural steps used in the meta-analysis of a nursing intervention research project, reflects those steps adapted from

Table 4
Procedural Steps of Meta-Analysis

1.0	Selection of the Question
	1.1 Formulation of a tentative question
	1.2 Specification of the methodological and substantive characteristics
	1.3 Development of a Glossary of Terms
	1.4 Refinement of the question(s)
2.0	Selection of the Data Space
	2.1 Specification of archival sources
	2.2 Specification of the sample of studies
	2.2.1 Development of criteria for inclusion/ exclusion
	2.2.2 Development of the list of key words
	2.2.3 Training of research assistants
	2.2.4 Construction of forms
	2.2.5 Title searches
	2.2.6 Intercoder agreements
	2.3 Specification of the potential corpus of studies
	2.4 Refinement of the conceptualization, glossary, and codebook elements
	2.4.1 Development of a classification scheme
	2.4.2 Development of an instrument for Quality of Study
3.0	Coding of Data
	3.1 Final decisions regarding eligibility into the corpus
	3.2 Retrieval of information for coding
	3.3 Obtaining intercoder agreements
	3.4 Further refinement of the codebook and glossary
4.0	Statistical treatment
	4.1 Computation of Chi-square and "z" corrected relative effect size per study and for the combined values (or effect consistent with the research question of the meta-analysis)
	4.2 Descriptive, multivariate, categorical, and group comparison statistics
5.0	Presentation and Analysis of Data
	5.1 Problem question results
	5.2 Elaboration of data regarding study characteristics
	5.3 Findings
6.0	Discussion, Conclusions, Implications, and Recommendations
	6.1 Conceptual framework
	6.2 Explanation of results
	6.3 Conclusions
	6.4 Recommendations
	6.4.1 Theory and research
	6.4.2 Research topics

recommendations by Glass, McGaw, and Smith (1981), Jackson (1980), Cooper (1982, 1984), and Light and Pillemer (1984). Clearly, meta-analysis is, for researchers, a rigorous research method, demanding strict protection against validity threats at each stage (Cooper, 1984).

Surrounding each step of the process are decision issues requiring explicit resolution. Detailed description of the conceptual and technical issues at hand are available in Smith (1987). Selected considerations are presented below.

Selection of the Question

Spencer (1860) questioned what knowledge was of most worth for practice. Building on this concern, Smith (1983) posed an even more fundamental issue: what is to count for knowledge itself? Because the question that inaugurates research arises out of a theoretical basis for the generation of nursing knowledge, the question, once formulated, and in the hierarchy of possible questions (Dillon, 1984), must also be consistent with available technology to provide meaningful results. For the researcher, it is the question that dictates the definition of study characteristics, the use of statistical treatment and meta-analysis formulas, and the characteristics of results.

For example, Devine and Cook (1983) performed a meta-analysis of studies to investigate the effect of psychoeducational interventions on postsurgical length of stay. They also posed the question of whether the effects of such interventions have remained stable over time despite the decrease in average length of stay. Through the selection of appropriate statistical methods their research provided not only a summary of the sampled studies, but also an estimate of the magnitude of and variations in the effect over time and across studies.

Selection of the Data Space

Researchers must identify and make explicit the nature of the information space (all possible sources of information) and the data space (sources for inclusion in the meta-analysis), as well as the rationale for source inclusion and exclusion (e.g., crossing of disciplines, only nurse-authored work, etc.). Those research designs most relevant to theory development may be an appropriate criterion here. To check for reliability, researchers must also identify the origin of lists of multiple sources of studies. For the researcher, the process generally moves from a large domain of possible titles, to the selection of a stratified random sample, to a potential corpus. From the latter, the researcher judges as appropriate for inclusion only those studies meeting the stringent criteria for the meta-analysis. The researcher then refines those elements begun in the first step of the meta-analysis so as to maintain internal consistency in the classification scheme, quality of study instrument, and codebook design.

Coding the Data

The researcher codes the data set, which consists of the study characteristics and the findings of each study, for the meta-analysis. These operationalized terms—data set, study characteristics, and findings—then represent the "conceived universe of discourse" (Mukherjee, 1983) for the project. The researcher can also assign each characteristic a level of abstraction consistent with the notions of distance from reality, as described by Maritain (1959), Reynolds (1971), and Rudner (1966). Here, the researcher should recognize the dangers of class and subclass data collapsing (Blalock, 1982), as well as the potential problems of rater "drift" as described by Orwin and Cordray (1985). As coding problems surface, they are resolved by the researcher through a rationale made explicit in the glossary of terms and procedures.

Statistical Treatment

The distance between conceptualization and measurement (Campbell, 1969) is an important issue when designing the statistical treatment appropriate for research questions. Mathematical foundations and assumptions underlie effect size equations and measurement manipulations. A variety of sources are available on statistical treatment in meta-analysis (Becker, 1987; Hedges & Olkin, 1985; Wolf, 1986). The researcher must reach decisions, for example, regarding the independence of outcomes across measures and what to do with outliers. Achieving a match between the research problem and appropriate statistical treatment is essential (Bangert-Drowns, 1986).

Presentation and Analysis of Data

The researcher uses traditional means of data illustration in meta-analysis with scrupulous attention to detail. In addition, the researcher often uses extended tables, figures, appendixes, and footnotes in meta-analysis reports.

Discussion, Conclusions, Implications, and Recommendations

The researcher should acknowledge that, while interpreting meta-analysis results, a *qualified* response to the research question has been generated. However, the researcher should acknowledge that only a *reduction*, not an elimination, of uncertainty (Shapiro, 1984) has been achieved.

Researchers also need to take into account the appropriateness of outcome indicators from conceptual, methodological, and pragmatic considerations. Researchers should recognize the importance of construct consistency within disciplines (Whitley, 1983), as well as construct validity in the primary research (Byrne, 1984; Shepard, Smith, & Vojir, 1983). Finally, researchers should recommend new primary studies to fill gaps, provide replications, vary situation specific circumstances, and entirely new meta-analyses to account for new perspectives.

CONCERNS

Each mathematical formula used in meta-analysis addresses a different question. Statistical treatment for meta-analysis is in a state of continuing refinement, demanding relentless updating with the literature. Consumers and researchers should be aware that currency with a methodology of such sophistication is essential. A meta-analysis project is probably best designed and implemented collaboratively by an interdisciplinary group of experts in the nursing phenomenon under study, meta-analysis, statistics, and computer technologies. Conceptualization of the phenomenon within the discipline of nursing also is critical to identification of study characteristics. Thus, the lack of nursing theory as the basis for dissertation and nursing intervention research reported in journals (Smith, 1988) weakens the scientific status of nursing knowledge as well as the validity of meta-analysis.

EVALUATION CRITERIA

A number of authors have recently proposed sets of criteria for evaluation of meta-analysis reports (Bangert-Drowns, 1986; Bullock & Svyantek, 1985; Light & Pillemer, 1984; Orwin & Cordray, 1985; Sacks et al., 1987). From these sources, the following criteria are suggested: (1) the purpose of the meta-analysis is made explicit; (2) use of a theoretical model serves as the basis of hypothesis testing, coding, and interpretation; (3) the basis for study selection is reported; (4) treatments in the studies are similar; (5) control groups are similar; (6) the unit of analysis is specified; (7) the distribution of outcomes is presented; (8) alternative explanations for findings are provided; (9) limits of generalizability are specified; and (10) sufficient detail of reporting is provided for replication.

THE FUTURE

Meta-analysis serves as a link between single studies and integration of these into the discipline. As a rigorous mode of inquiry to consolidate multiple studies into a unified whole, meta-analysis approaches contribute to theory development. The results of meta-analysis generate new hypotheses for testing, make state-of-the-art descriptions of phenomena and their properties derived from research bases, and reveal gaps in the literature. Meta-analysis projects provide replicable and credible bases for findings. The cataloging of phenomena essential to science (Rudner, 1966) also emerges as a by-product of meta-analysis. The application of the research process to a collection of studies has the potential to transform discrete bits of *information* into the *knowledge* of a discipline.

REFERENCES

Axelson, M. L., Federline, T. L., & Brinberg, D. (1985). A meta-analysis of food- and nutrition-related research. *Journal of Nutrition Education, 17*(2), 51–54.

Bangert-Drowns, R. L. (1986). Review of developments in meta-analytic method. *Psychological Bulletin, 99*, 388–399.

Becker, B. J. (1987). Applying tests of combined significance in meta-analysis. *Psychological Bulletin, 102*, 164–171.

Black, M. (1954). *Problems of analysis: Philosophical essays.* Ithaca: Cornell University Press.

Blalock, H. M. (1982). *Conceptualization and measurement in the social sciences.* Beverly Hills: Sage Publications.

Blalock, H. M. (1984). *Basic dilemmas in the social sciences.* Beverly Hills: Sage Publications.

Booth-Kewley, S., & Friedman, H. S. (1987). Psychological predictors of heart disease: A quantitative review. *Psychological Bulletin, 101*, 343–359.

Bullock, R. J., & Svyantek, D. J. (1985). Analyzing meta-analyses: Potential problems, an unsuccessful replication and evaluation criteria. *Journal of Applied Psychology, 70*, 108–115.

Byrne, B. M. (1984). The general/academic self-concept nomological network: A review of construct validation research. *Review of Educational Research, 54*, 427–456.

Campbell, D. T. (1969). Definitional versus multiple operationism. *Et Al.*, *2*, 14–17.

Cochran, W. G. (1937). Problems arising in the analysis of a series of similar experiments. *Journal of the Royal Statistical Society*, *4* (Suppl.), 102–118.

Colton, T., Freedman, L. S., & Johnson, A. L. (Eds.). (1987). *Statistics in medicine* (Vol. 6, No. 3). New York: Wiley.

Cooper, H. M. (1982). Scientific guidelines for conducting integrative research reviews. *Review of Educational Research*, *52*, 291–302.

Cooper, H. M. (1984). *The integrative research review: A systematic approach.* Beverly Hills: Sage Publications.

Dagenais, J. J. (1972). *Models of man: A phenomenological critique of some paradigms in the human sciences.* The Hague, Netherlands: Martinus Nijhoff.

Devine, E. C., & Cook, T. D. (1983). A meta-analytic analysis of effects of psychoeducational interventions on length of post-surgical hospital stay. *Nursing Research*, *32*, 267–274.

Dewey, J. (1938). *Experience and education.* New York: Collier Books.

Dillon, J. T. (1984). The classification of research questions. *Review of Educational Research*, *54*, 327–361.

Falbo, T., & Polit, D. (1985). A meta-analysis of the only child literature. *Pediatric Nursing*, *11*, 356–360.

Fisher, R. A. (1932). *Statistical methods for research workers* (4th ed.). London: Oliver and Boyd.

Friedman, H. S., & Booth-Kewley, S. (1987). The disease-prone personality: A meta-analytic view of the construct. *American Psychologist*, *42*, 539–555.

Garfield, S. L. (1983). Meta-analysis and psychotherapy [Special section]. *Journal of Consulting and Clinical Psychology*, *51*(1).

Glass, G. V., McGaw, B., & Smith, M. L. (1981). *Meta-analysis in social research.* Beverly Hills: Sage Publications.

Haring-Hidore, M., et al. (1985). Marital status and subjective well-being. *Journal of Marriage and the Family*, *47*, 947–953.

Harré, R. (1972). *The philosophies of science.* Oxford: Oxford University Press.

Hedges, L. V., & Olkin, I. (1985). *Statistical methods for meta-analysis.* Orlando, FL: Academic Press, Inc.

Hendrick, C., & Jones, R. A. (1972). *The nature of theory and research in social psychology.* New York: Academic Press.

Hidi, S., & Anderson, V. (1986). Producing written summaries: Task demands, cognitive operations, and implications for instruction. *Review of Educational Research*, *56*, 473–493.

Hull, J. G., & Bond, C. F. (1986). Social and behavioral consequences of alcohol-consumption and expectancy: A meta-analysis. *Psychological Bulletin*, *99*, 347–360.

Hunter, J. E., Schmidt, F. L., & Jackson, G. B. (1982). *Meta-analysis: Cumulating research findings across studies.* Beverly Hills: Sage Publications.

Jackson, G. B. (1980). Methods for integrative reviews. *Review of Educational Research, 50*, 438–460.

Janicak, P. G., Davis, J. M., Gibbons, R. D., Ericksen, S., Chang, S., & Gallagher, P. C. (1985). Efficacy of ECT: A meta-analysis. *American Journal of Psychiatry, 142*, 297–302.

Johnson, D. W., & Johnson, R. T. (1985). Nutrition education: A model for effectiveness, a synthesis of research. *Journal of Nutrition Education, 17* (Suppl. June), S11–S19, S25–S44.

Jones, L. C. (1983). *A meta-analytic study of childbirth education research from 1960-1981.* Unpublished doctoral dissertation, Texas A & M University, College Station.

Kulik, J. A., Kulik, C. L. C., & Cohen, P. A. (1979). A meta-analysis of outcome studies of Keller's personalized system of instruction. *American Psychologist, 34*, 307–318.

Light, R. J., & Pillemer, D. B. (1984). *Summing up: The science of reviewing research.* Cambridge, MA: Harvard University Press.

Lonergan, B. (1980). *Understanding and being: An introduction and companion to insight.* New York: The Edwin Mellen Press.

Louis, T. A., Fineberg, H. V., & Mosteller, F. (1985). Findings for public health from meta-analysis. *Annual Review of Public Health, 6*, 1–20.

Lynn, D. D., & Donovan, J. M. (1980). Medical versus surgical treatment of coronary artery disease. *Evaluation in Education: An International Review Series, 4*(1), 98–99.

Maritain, J. (1959). *The degrees of knowledge* (G. B. Phelan, Trans.). New York: Charles Scribner's Sons.

Michelson, L. (Ed.). (1985). Meta-analysis and clinical psychology. *Clinical Psychology Review, 5*(1).

Mukherjee, R. (1983). *Classification in social research.* Albany: State University of New York Press.

Mullen, P. D., Green, L. W., & Persinger, G. S. (1985). Clinical trials of patient education for chronic conditions: A comparative meta-analysis of intervention types. *Preventive Medicine, 14*, 753–781.

Mumford, E., Schlesinger, H. J., & Glass, G. V. (1982). The effects of psychological intervention on recovery from surgery and heart attacks: An analysis of the literature. *American Journal of Public Health, 72*, 141–151.

Munevar, G. (1981). *Radical knowledge: A philosophical inquiry into the nature and limits of science.* Indianapolis: Hackett Publishing Co.

Nunes, E. V., & Frank, K. A., & Kornfeld, D. S. (1986). Psychological treatment for coronary prone behavior: A meta-analysis of the literature. *Psychosomatic Medicine, 48*, 306.

Orwin, R. G., & Cordray, D. S. (1985). Effects of deficient reporting on meta-analysis: A conceptual framework and reanalysis. *Psychological Bulletin, 97*, 134–147.

Pearson, K. (1933). On a method of determining whether a sample of size n, supposed to have been drawn from a parent population having a known probability integral, has probably been drawn at random. *Biometrika, 25,* 379–410.

Posavac, E. J. (1980). Evaluation of patient education programs: A meta-analysis. *Evaluation and the Health Professions, 3,* 47–62.

Reynolds, P. D. (1971). *A primer in theory construction.* Indianapolis: The Bobbs-Merrill Company.

Rosenthal, R. (1984). *Meta-analytic procedures for social research.* Beverly Hills: Sage Publications.

Rotton, J., & Kelly, I. W. (1985). Much ado about the full moon: A meta-analysis of lunar-lunacy research. *Psychological Bulletin, 97,* 286–306.

Rudner, R. S. (1966). *Philosophy of social science.* Englewood Cliffs, NJ: Prentice-Hall.

Sacks, H. S., Berrier, J., Reitman, D., Ancona-Berk, V. A., & Chalmers, T. C. (1987). Meta-analyses of randomized controlled trials. *The New England Journal of Medicine, 316,* 450–455.

Schwartz, R., Moody, L., Yarandi, H., & Anderson, G. C. (1987). A meta-analysis of critical outcome variables in nonnutritive sucking in preterm infants. *Nursing Research, 36,* 292–295.

Shapiro, J. Z. (1984). On the application of econometric methodology to educational research: A meta-theoretical analysis. *Educational Researcher, 13*(2), 12–19.

Shepard, L. A., Smith, M. L., & Vojir, C. P. (1983). Characteristics of pupils identified as learning disabled. *American Educational Research Journal, 20,* 309–331.

Smith, J. K. (1983). Quantitative versus qualitative research: An attempt to clarify the issue. *Educational Researcher, 12*(3), 6–13.

Smith, M. C. (1987). Meta-analysis: Conceptual issues. In S. R. Gortner (Ed.), *Nursing science methods: A reader.* San Francisco: Regents, University of California, pp. 59–76.

Smith, M. C. (1988). *Meta-analysis of nursing intervention research.* Birmingham: Birmingham Printing and Publishing Company.

Smith, M. C., & Naftel, D. C. (1984). Meta-analysis: A perspective for research synthesis. *Image: The Journal of Nursing Scholarship, 16*(1), 9–13.

Spencer, H. (1860). What knowledge is of most worth? In *Education.* New York: Appleton-Century-Crofts.

Stevenson, M. R. (1985). *The effects of paternal absence on sex-role development: A meta-analysis.* Unpublished doctoral dissertation, Purdue University.

Stock, W. A., Okun, M. A., Haring, M. H., Miller, W., Kinney, C., & Ceurvorst, R. W. (1982). Rigor in data synthesis: A case of reliability in meta-analysis. *Educational Researcher, 11*(6), 10–14, 20.

Straw, R. B. (1983). Deinstitutionalization in mental health: A meta-analysis. In R. J. Light (Ed.), *Evaluation studies: Review Annual* (Vol. 8, pp. 253–278). Beverly Hills: Sage Publications.

Suppe, F. (Ed.). (1974). *The structure of scientific theories.* Urbana, IL: University of Illinois Press.

Thomas, J. R., & French, K. E. (1986). The use of meta-analysis in exercise and sport: A tutorial. *Research Quarterly For Exercise and Sport, 57,* 196–204.

Tippett, L. H. C. (1931). *The methods of statistics.* London: Williams and Norgate.

Turley, M. A. (1985). A meta-analysis of informing mothers concerning the sensory and perceptual capabilities of their infants: The effects on maternal-infant interaction. *Maternal Child Nursing, 14,* 183–197.

Vance, E. C. (1986). *Correlates of mother-infant attachment: A meta-analysis.* Unpublished doctoral dissertation. Texas A & M University, College Station.

Wampler, K. (1982). Bringing the review of literature into the age of quantification: Meta-analyses as a strategy for integrating research findings in family studies. *Journal of Marriage and the Family, 44,* 1009–1023.

Whitley, B. E. (1983). Sex role orientation and self-esteem: A critical meta-analytic review. *Journal of Personality and Social Psychology, 44,* 765–778.

Wolf, F. M. (1986). *Meta-analysis: Quantitative methods for research synthesis.* Beverly Hills: Sage Publications.

Part 2
The Personal Path
to Nursing Knowledge

In contrast to empirical modes of inquiry, personal modes focus on subjective rather than objective experience. Phenomenology, though often classed with ethnography and grounded theory as a qualitative method, is distinguished from these two on this point. The subjective experience of informants is not excluded from ethnography and grounded theory, but it is not the *primary* concern of the inquiry as in phenomenology. The subject matter of phenomenology is the lived experience of individuals, with the goal of describing and understanding subjectively encountered human conditions or events such as pain, courage, cancer, or miscarriage. Generalizations are made by inductive methods, yet these generalizations maintain their focus on personal experience.

The development of personal ways of knowing is an exciting and significant step in the evolution of nursing. Nursing scholars are acknowledging the value and central role of the individual and of the nurse/patient encounter. Other research methods under development in the personal mode of inquiry include case studies and transcendental phenomenology. The reader is challenged to reflect on the richness and depth of meaning to be found in this path to nursing knowledge.

Phenomenology

Kristen Swanson-Kauffman and Elizabeth Schonwald

Phenomenology is both a philosophical movement and a research methodology (Cohen, 1987). As a philosophy, phenomenology deals in the realm of the ideal, pure, and perfect. As a methodology, it deals in the practical world of concession, compromise, and approximation. The reason for this seeming contradiction is that phenomenological philosophers strive to articulate a coherent and cohesive description of existence, of "being-in-the-world." Phenomenological researchers strive to understand and describe lived experiences.

As a philosophical movement of the nineteenth century, phenomenology has had a profound impact on how nurses and other scientists view the nature of being in the world. Such influence is obvious in the proliferation of qualitative methodologies now employed by scientists in the late twentieth century. Grounded theory, phenomenology, ethnomethodology, and ethnography are among the methodologies which were supported by the philosophy of science current during the nineteenth-century's period of Enlightenment. Each of these strategies involves a discipline—a specific attempt to enact a methodology which would allow investigators to rigorously apprehend experiences as they are perceived by those individuals, groups, or societies who live them.

Nursing, especially in the last 15 years, has become increasingly committed to the appropriateness of the various qualitative methodologies for the study of nursing phenomena. Since nursing practice involves diagnosing and treating human responses to actual and potential health problems, and since humans respond as whole persons, knowledge of the lived experiences of health and healing are legitimate topics of nursing inquiry.

This chapter will examine phenomenology as a method for nursing research. In reviewing several interpretations of the phenomenological method (Colaizzi, 1978; Giorgi, 1970; Marton & Svensson, 1979), we have observed four basic strategies inherent in each method. These strategies—bracketing, analyzing, intuiting, and describing—may be summarized as the four essential steps in "getting back to the things themselves." We will use these four basic steps as a framework for describing our own experiences with phenomenological inquiry. Futhermore, we will relate these four basic steps to Carper's (1978) description of the four ways of knowing in nursing (ethical, esthetic, empirical, and personal knowledge). Within each of the steps and ways of knowing we will use examples from our own studies in order to highlight how we have carried out phenomenological inquiry in designing and implementing nursing studies.

BRACKETING: THE ETHICS OF PHENOMENOLOGY

Edmund Husserl is credited with establishing the fundamental principle of phenomenology. His expression, "back to the things themselves," is recognized as the guiding theme for phenomenological research (Omery, 1983). According to Giorgi (1985), Husserl's continuing appeal is in his recognition of the importance and value of returning to the everyday world "where people are living through various phenomena in actual situations" (p. 8). The imperative to turn to the people who actually live the experience is, in effect, the "should," or the ethical dictum, of phenomenology. The imperative to accurately interpret lived experiences is the phenomenological researcher's guiding principle. In fact, the very worth of a phenomenological portrayal of reality must be judged in terms of how validly the researcher represents the experiences of those who live the reality.

Bracketing, the setting aside of researcher assumptions both prior to and during the actual data gathering, is the methodological attempt to accurately portray the reality of informants. Through bracketing, the researcher attempts to reduce her own assumptions about the reality of the phenomenon studied. A second layer of bracketing involves, prior to and during each interview, reducing the influence of the witness of all previous informants in order to fully heed the story of the one who is being queried. Always a problematic task, bracketing is an attempt to bridge the gap between the researcher's own experience of the phenomenon studied and the reality that exists outside of the investigator's personal world. In effect, bracketing is the tool used to meet the ethical dictum of portraying accurately the reality of the phenomenon as it is lived and described by the researcher's informants.

For our work, we have translated bracketing in this manner: It is a concerted attempt to negotiate the empirical with the experiential. Because phenomenological inquiry is a process with unclear beginning, conclusion, and a continuous effort to reconcile personal knowledge and beliefs with the witness of informants, several leaps of faith are necessary. First, we must believe that our experiences and knowledge, while valid, may not be the reality of those we seek to describe. Second, we must believe that we are capable of eliciting and hearing the reality of our informants. Third, we must believe that the personal stories of our informants will express a reality sufficiently unique or cohesive so that any a priori assumptions of our own will not influence their interpretation.

However, because it is we who have raised research questions, we cannot help but express opinions about that which we believe is worth studying. For example, in 1986 Swanson-Kauffman conducted research on parents' experiences in the neonatal intensive care unit (NICU); she had initiated that study based on her own son's brief NICU admission. Furthermore, as with any other study, her phenomenological research proposal had to be submitted to scientific review boards, ethics committees, and funding agencies. Personal experiences, literature searches, and review boards' comments all contribute to any researcher's a priori assumptions about the reality of the phenomenon investigated.

Yet several ways exist in which we try to bracket our experiential knowledge of the phenomenon studied in order to "capture" the empirical reality outside of ourselves. First, it is necessary to state clearly our conscious assumptions about that which we are investigating. This step also serves the needs of review agencies to see that our study is grounded in a real world. The articulation of personal assumptions, in a traditional research proposal, takes the place of the conceptual framework section. Within those assumptions, we state the beliefs we presently hold about the answer to the research question and identify which theories or research studies we believe are salient to the question posed. Although to some phenomenological researchers the fact that we do a literature review may seem like heresy, we believe that it is a practical concession to the realities of the research world. We also believe that the research done by others and the clinical and lay articles that we review before interviewing research subjects are legitimate attempts to bracket our own personal biases by examining others' descriptions of empirical instances of the phenomenon under study.

ANALYZING: THE EMPIRICS OF PHENOMENOLOGY

The rigorous gathering and analyzing of interview data constitute the empirical aspect of the phenomenological study. This is the phase of inquiry in which the researcher attempts to gather accounts of lived experiences of a phenomenon. The researcher, having bracketed personal beliefs about the reality of the queried phenomenon, strives to systematically gather data beyond her personal experiences. In effect, the empirics of phenomenology involve establishing a plan through which data may be located, gathered, recorded, sorted, retrieved, condensed, and verified.

In our studies, the empirical phase begins with identification of the population from which subjects will be selected. The population is chosen for its members' experience with the phenomenon or condition of interest. The actual subjects are selected in order to maximize the potential for achieving as much variability in accounts of the phenomenon as possible.

Subsequent to specifying the desired population, the phenomenological researcher generates a tentative interview schedule. The schedule serves only as a prompting device. The types of questions included are meant to be provocative and creative means of getting informants to talk about their own experiences of the phenomenon. Between each planned question, therefore, the interviewer's goal is to keep the informant talking about events and their meaning.

We are most comfortable recording our data via a taperecording of interviews. The recordings are subsequently transcribed verbatim. When appropriate, *The Ethnograph* (Seidel, Kjolseth, & Seymour, 1988), a software package used for qualitative data analysis, is used as a means of storing and retrieving data. In 1986, Swanson-Kauffman elaborated on one means of using *The Ethnograph* to discretely code the experience of a limited ($n = 20$) number of *like* subjects speaking to a specific experience (i.e., miscarriage). She has since discovered that the discrete, concise coding of all lines of every subject's data can not and does not make sense for every phenomenological study. For example, in her study of caring in the NICU, several different types of care providers (mothers, fathers, nurses, and physicians) were interrogated about their experiences of providing and receiving care in the NICU. Each subject's story was so tied to his role that a cross-subject line by line coding schema became unwieldy, cumbersome, and stifling. In the NICU study, analysis required a more creative attempt to answer the question, "Given all these different stories, what ultimately do these providers have in common?"

Multiple readings and rereadings of entire transcripts and comparisons among persons and events; discussions with subjects and research colleagues; multiple free-writings (see Elbow, 1986); and a tremendous amount of reflective self-talk ultimately led to a theoretical model of providing care in the NICU. In this study, concise coding was a detraction that led the investigator away from the more productive intuitive aspects of inquiry.

Once the model is generated, the task of verification follows. This may take several forms. In Schonwald's (1988) study of the experiences of interpreters in the health care system, verification took two main forms: internal and external. Internal verification included: returning to subjects for a second interview to see if their stories were consistent with their first interview and to get the subject's critique of the credibility of the emerging theoretical model; and reanalyzing each subject's transcript while noting and critiquing the applicability of each category to each subject. External verification of Schonwald's model included: reexamining the original assumptions and comparing her model to other descriptions of experiences of interpreters (both within the health care system and on the local and international scenes); and comparing and contrasting her phases of the experience of interpreters to Swanson-Kauffman's (1988) caring concepts.

INTUITING: THE PERSONAL LINK TO THE OTHER'S REALITY

Reinharz (1984) refers to qualitative research as a three-pronged challenge consisting of understanding the substantive problem studied; allowing personal change to occur, especially on the part of the investigator; and creating innovative methodological strategies to capture the unique features of each project. The key to each of these challenges is a researcher who is willing to operate in a methodology that mandates an investment of the personal self in the topic investigated. Unlike a positivistic paradigm that values distance and objectivity, the outcome of phenomenological inquiry depends on the researcher's ability to engage with the informants' reality. Such engagement does not mean that the investigator has to have lived the phenomenon studied; rather it means the investigator must approach each informant's story with an empathic sense. Noddings (1984), in discussing caring, captures the experience of intuiting another's reality by saying the one who cares strives to understand "as if"—as if the other's reality were her own. The phenomenological researcher intuits the other's reality by being open to identifying with the other's self and considering the other's reality as a possible reality for herself.

As stated earlier, the researcher must identify a means of locating a population that has witnessed the phenomenon of interest and a strategy for assisting the chosen sample to describe their experience with the phenomenon. Because informants must speak freely and reflectively about experiences that may not be easy to discuss, the researcher must help them dig deeply into thoughts that may not be a part of their everyday awareness. This type of data soliciting demands that the researcher move into a mode of being that is (1) hyperattentive to the informant's words and gestures; (2) totally believing that the informant is an expert on the topic of inquiry by virtue of the fact that he has lived his own experience of the phenomenon studied; and (3) on-the-spot creative in assisting the informant to reflect on the meaning of events as they are discussed. Such hyperattentiveness, belief, and creativity are all reliant on the researcher's self engaging in the data-gathering process. In effect, the researcher's role is to move back and forth between intuiting and verifying with the informant as the informant's story unfolds. The intellectual and emotional challenges of qualitative inquiry are captured by Johnson (1975) in his discussion of Bergson's beliefs about intuiting:

> Now it is clear that any new advance . . . demands a method that can give us direct access to internal organization and existential reality of phenomena themselves. Bergson argues that intuition is the only method of investigation that can provide us such direct access to the mystery of existence and to the absolute nature of reality. He means by intuition a kind of "intellectual sympathy" by which one places oneself within an object in order to coincide with what is unique in it. (p. 229)

We have discovered over time that the marks of good qualitative interview are: (1) if at the end of the interview, the client replies to the question, "Is there anything more about your experience with (the phenomenon) that you believe is important and that we may not have touched on?" with the response "No way, you actually got me talking about feelings about (the phenomenon) that I wasn't even aware I was feeling."; and (2) if the client immediately or weeks later says, "Thank you, that really helped me to make sense of the whole experience." It did take us some getting used to the fact that informants often confused phenomenological research data gathering with a caring therapeutic encounter. However, we have come to accept this as hardly surprising. Rarely do any of us experience the opportunity to feel so genuinely understood by another person as with the authentic openness that is part of the qualitative method.

In a qualitative interview, the researcher also changes for the encounter. Breaking into and, for the time, experiencing another's reality, leads the researcher to awareness of how similar or different the other's reality is to hers. When a similarity in feeling exists, the researcher, without having disclosed her own thoughts, also feels understood. When the informant's reality is markedly dissimilar, the researcher continues to experience insight into her own beliefs because of the contrast in life experiences.

A final aspect of intuiting that causes concern is in how the researcher moves from data (multiple informants' accounts of their reality of the phenomenon) to a presentation of a summary of the phenomenon (most often in the form of a theoretical model of the phenomenon and its component processes). In truth, this is very hard to say. It is like trying to say how you know when you know something *and* when you first knew that you knew it. Intuiting concepts of the final model is an exercise that involves continuous critical reflection and discussion of concepts as they emerge from the researcher's experience of the multiple informants' reality. Such reflection involves internal struggle wherein the researcher wonders, "How could it be that these diverse, unique stories are discussing the same phenomena? What processes might embrace these contrary situations and reduce them to a conceptual level that accounts for their apparent diversity?" Discussion involves going to other qualitative researchers and asking them to help you resolve internal struggles or to validate the soundness of hypothesized categories. Although others may not have been part of the inquiry, an attentive critic can offer invaluable perspective in helping to make sense of emergent thoughts.

As in the qualitative interview itself, the intuitive phase of analysis demands that the researcher be hyperattentive to her own thoughts and feelings about the data. Furthermore, the researcher must achieve a balance between being too critical and too accepting of her beliefs about emerging concepts. The researcher must believe that the phenomenon can be grasped and that she will see the phenomenon and its processes if a vigilant attempt is made to balance the expanding experiential with the incoming empirical. When a phenomenon is finally understood, and its processes or categories identified, the researcher will find that new, incoming, empirical data will seem to fit or be subsumed under the now-defined categories. Being able to fit problematic situations under previously identified concepts is the hallmark of a saturated description of a phenomenon.

DESCRIBING: THE ESTHETICS OF PHENOMENOLOGICAL INQUIRY

There is an art to phenomenological inquiry. The researcher must approach the subjects and subject matter with a sense of awe, empathy, and appreciation. The techniques for the conduct of inquiry are very difficult to describe or write about. It is best conveyed to a novice through example, coaching, and constructive critique. While it is rigorous, it is not rigid. There must be a self-imposed discipline and structure to bridge the gaps between data collection, intuition, and ultimate description of the salient concepts. Because phenomenology relies so heavily on the investigator's disciplined attempt to personally enter into the reality of others, it is difficult to *prescribe* how that is to be done. Creativity and a willingness to take chances are often times the phenomenological investigator's only keys to entering, sharing, and reporting on the reality of others.

A model derived from phenomenological inquiry can and should be esthetically appealing. While a well-done model should be universal enough to apply to each informant, it should also be simple and straightforward. A phenomenological model is like a universal skeleton that can be filled in with the rich story of each informant. The model will not account for the complete story of each informant; yet it should be applicable to each informant. If the investigator has truly identified the components (also called processes, parts, or categories) of a phenomenon, then anyone who has experienced the phenomenon should be able to analyze their own reality with the identified components.

CONCLUSION

In this chapter, we have equated Carper's (1978) four fundamental patterns of knowing in nursing with the four basic steps of phenomenology. Although we have associated each phenomenological step with a pattern of knowing, we have also set arbitrary boundaries around each step of the phenomenological process. We believe that just as true understanding in a clinical moment is the result of a simultaneous experience of all four patterns of knowing, so too is each moment in the phenomenological investigation a blend of bracketing, analyzing, intuiting, and describing.

REFERENCES

Carper, B. A. (1978). Fundamental patterns of knowing in nursing. *Advances in Nursing Science, 1*, 13–23.

Cohen, M. Z. (1987). A historical overview of the phenomenological movement. *Image*, 19, 31–34.

Colaizzi, P. F. (1978). Psychological research as the phenomenologist views it. In R. Vaile & M. King (Eds.), *Existential phenomenological alternatives for psychology*. New York: Oxford University Press.

Elbow, P. (1986). *Embracing contraries*. New York: Oxford University Press.

Giorgi, A. (1970). *Psychology as a human science: A phenomenologically based approach*. New York: Harper & Row.

Giorgi, A. (1985). *Phenomenology and psychological research*. Pittsburgh: Duquesne University Press.

Johnson, R. E. (1975). *In quest of a new psychology*. New York: Human Sciences Press.

Marton, F., & Svensson, L. (1979). Concepts of research in student learning. *Higher Education, 8*, 471–486.

Noddings, N. (1984). *Caring: A feminine approach to ethics and moral education*. Berkeley: University of California Press.

Omery, A. (1983). Phenomenology: A method for nursing research. *Advances in Nursing Science, 5*, 49–63.

Reinharz, S. (1984). *On becoming a social scientist: From survey research and participant observation to experiential analysis*. New Brunswick, NJ: Transaction Books, p. xi.

Schonwald, E. (1988). *The experience of interpreters within the health care system*. Unpublished master's thesis, University of Washington, Seattle, WA.

Seidel, J., Kjolseth, R., & Seymour, E. (1988). *The Ethnograph*. Littleton, CO: Qualis Research Associates.

Swanson-Kauffman, K. M. (1986). A combined qualitative methodology for nursing research. *Advances in Nursing Science, 8*, 58–69.

Swanson-Kauffman, K. M. (1988). Empirical development and refinement of a model of caring. Abstract in *Communicating Nursing Research, 21*, 80.

Part 3
The Esthetic Path
to Nursing Knowledge

Esthetic research offers unlimited opportunity for creativity and richness of meaning in the expression of nursing knowledge. The chapter illustrating this path describes the utilization of photodocumentation as a research method. Esthetic paths focus on a single moment in time, a discrete bit of experience in the domain of nursing, creatively and imaginatively expressed. Literature, poetry, art, music, dance, drama, photography, cinema—all hold tremendous potential for providing nurse researchers with a wealth of meaningful data. In the last few years, scattered pieces of artistic expression have appeared in the nursing literature, an exciting development which can be expected to further inspire a freeing of creative energy within the discipline.

Esthetic Inquiry

Betty Highley and Tom Ferentz

When I first became interested in photography . . . my idea was to have it recognized as one of the fine arts. Today, I don't give a hoot in hell about that. The mission of photography is to explain man to man and each man to himself. And that is the most complicated thing on earth and also as naive as a tender plant. . .

Edward Steichen (Capa, 1972)

In 1981, when we established Visual Media Research, our desire was to explore the relationship between the sciences and arts through photography in order to further extend our knowledge of clinical interactions and human behavior. The process we describe in this chapter is an adaptation of the historic tradition of documentary photography and the scientific method. Through the practice of photography and the analysis of photographs, we have attempted to add another dimension of truthfulness to the reconstruction and reporting of our observations and to the sharpening of our visual senses. Our overriding purpose remains now as it did then—to communicate and educate.

One of the more subtle aspects of our work has been to reassert humanistic and compassionate dimensions of health care; dimensions which are seriously endangered by the demands of a highly technological field. Hopefully, a newly sensitized awareness of the clinical environment can be achieved through viewing and studying visual data by way of the photographic image.

Research relies on collecting, recording, and analyzing information. At a minimum, the camera can serve as a notebook for recording visual content to facilitate more objective recollection on the part of the re-searcher/observer. Through the analysis of visual recordings, significant-

111

ly more data can be obtained than through notes, tape recordings, and memory alone. Considering the facility with which photographs lend themselves to communication, it is remarkable that within the health sciences—where need for continued exploration of communications exists—relatively little attention has been given to visual literacy in the education and preparation of health professionals and researchers. Because of this, a primary function of the visual media program is teaching nurses to use cameras in their clinical practice and research.

From the time nurses enter into their professional education and throughout their careers, they must constantly sophisticate their skills in observing and listening. Once one has seen and heard, it becomes necessary to reconstruct the information and pass it on to others. This reconstruction is dependent on accuracy of recall.

It is significant to note that we oftentimes lack complete confidence in what was said. We are concerned that we may hear what we want to hear or what we think is being said. We are constantly processing what is said through our own biases and experiences. Thus, we use a tape recorder to ensure an accurate record.

On the other hand, we place far more confidence in our ability to recall that which we see. However, we process what we see through the same veil of personal experiences and understandings we have grown to mistrust in our ears. There is an old saying: "The eyes believe themselves, the ears believe other people." If we acknowledge this as an inconsistency in our attitudes toward sensory data, then the camera presents itself as the obvious instrument for recording visual information, just as the tape recorder is used for sound.

Examples and anecdotes of clinicians sensing that a patient is going bad, or that there is a change in their status, abound. This process, which relies on a complex synthesis of what are often extremely subtle non-verbal cues, is difficult to articulate. Through the study of this process of clinical assessment, Benner (1984) has developed the concept of "perceptual knowledge." How do we find the words which describe this perceptual knowledge to enable us to teach, communicate, and pass it on to others?

This chapter includes background on research using visual media, including models from the social sciences and photography. Issues related to methodology and design are discussed, and suggestions for the use of photography in nursing research are presented.

BACKGROUND AND HISTORICAL PERSPECTIVE

Anthropology and sociology are two disciplines that make extensive use of photo documentation. In 1986, John Collier authored the first text on visual research, *Visual Anthropology: Photography as a Research Method*, addressing issues of anthropological fieldwork.

Collier's book contains a statement on research procedure and a treatise on observation and interpretation. Though addressed to anthropologists, Collier's book has become the primary model for all of the behavioral sciences in which the recording and interpretation of visual data are significant.

While we credit Collier for promoting photography in both the academic and research settings, Margret Mead was the first to use photography in her own research. Published in 1942, *Balinese Character*, although a controversial work, is her classic study done in 1936–1939. Her then husband, Gregory Bateson, took the photographs while Mead made observations and wrote field notes. The sequential photographs accompanied by her voluminous notes on each frame contributed to what is perhaps the most ambitious piece of anthropological fieldwork ever published. Included were 759 photographs arranged on 100 sequential plates accompanied by Mead's detailed, on the spot, notes. One methodological issue which evolves out of this work is the separation of visual recorder and observer/interviewer.

Within the last decade, a number of sociologists have begun to use photography as a research tool. Howard Becker, a distinguished professor at Northwestern University in Illinois, has provided significant leadership in this area. In 1981, Becker organized a major traveling exhibition, "Exploring Society Photographically," which surveyed the uses of photography in the social sciences. This exhibition and its accompanying book have had an appreciable impact on documentary photography in the visual arts as well as on the social sciences.

One of the most prominent examples of a photographer whose concerns relate to the health sciences is photojournalist, W. Eugene Smith. Originally a war photographer, Smith saw the period after World War II as an opportunity for journalism to apply itself to something other than the sensationalist coverage of wartime reportage. Integral to his view of journalism was an extraordinary conception of a role for photography. It was based on an appreciation for the communicative potential of photographs. Using photographs, not text, as a basis for writing stories, Smith developed the form of the photo essay while working for Life magazine (Johnson, 1981).

Smith's methodology bore striking similarities to anthropological field research. He spent a great deal of time with his subjects, developing close relationships with them to better tell stories. He broke with the journalistic tradition by developing a style that focused on the *intent* of the activity. In a non-intrusive way, he photographed elements of a scene that defined its content.

Two of Smith's photo-essays of particular significance to the health sciences are "The Country Doctor" and "Nurse-Midwife." In these two photo essays, Smith followed his subjects through their daily activities working in rural communities. The nurse-midwife, for example, as the only full-time caregiver in her area, is shown performing a variety of services. Smith's photographs of her could serve as a guideline for many specializations in the field of nursing. We must also note that Smith's "Nurse-Midwife" story stimulated donations of funds sufficient to build a clinic for the nurse-midwife. Unfortunately, however, "Nurse-Midwife" is a historical document of a way to provide health care that is rapidly disappearing.

Visual statements like Smith's teach us about the effects of nurses and doctors working *with* people. Rather than show us how to perform a particular skilled function, they speak about how and under what circumstances care is given.

In the mid-1960s, Highley (1967) conducted a one-year research study on maternal role identity with a small group of young mothers and their firstborn infants. At the conclusion of the study, Highley photographed some of the subjects. Each mother and infant were requested to pose in whatever way was most comfortable without any arranging or suggesting by Highley. When Highley showed the photographs to a group of post-master's students and colleagues, they were able to accurately describe each mother's patterns of response to her infant and to draw conclusions about the mothering style and maternal–infant interactions. In short, they were able to summarize research that had been gleaned over a one-year period. This pointed the way to more direct uses of photography in nursing research.

METHODOLOGICAL AND DESIGN ISSUES

Purpose and Framework

Before undertaking a visual documentation project, the researcher must clearly understand its purpose. To what end are the photographs being taken? What is their intent? The purposes may range from the microscopic analysis of non-verbal communications of an infant with a tracheotomy to a macroscopic analysis of environmental inventories. Consideration must be given to the visibility of the elements central to the problem.

Second, the framework out of which visual documentation evolves must be clearly understood. More often than not, the philosophical stance and theoretical underpinnings are more implicit then explicit. Such implicit aspects in the approach of an individual practitioner or researcher to his or her subjects will influence the photography. Further, we have discovered that the process of photographing often leads to a rigorous self-examination. As a result, misconceptions and a priori beliefs become known to the researcher—an advantage that is always of great value to a more comprehensive understanding of the subjects or phenomenon under study.

Design issues are as varied as are the problems and purposes being addressed. Additionally, it should be emphasized that we are not discussing a tool that is a panacea to all non-verbal data collection. Rather, it is a tool which, like the tape recorder, can make a significant contribution in our search for knowledge.

Access and Consent

We use two approaches in the design of projects: the case study and the agency or service survey. In the latter approach, systematic fact-finding precedes the actual work of visual documentation. First and foremost, however, are issues of access and consent. While these have the potential to get complicated, it is significant that over a period of six years, both in our own and in our student's work, we have encountered only a limited number of refusals to sign a release and give consent. In fact, we have been more excited by the dynamics suggested by subjects not only in consenting, but who appear to want to have a photo taken. There is also increasing evidence that the process of visually recording has, in some cases, a therapeutic effect (Higgens & Highley, 1986).

Agency access is another matter, and is often dependent on how sensitive to visual communications the director is and how confident and even proud he or she is of the agency's service. The agency's forms often include a consent and release for photographs. However, it must be stressed that regardless of blanket consent, no photograph is ever taken without verbal consent on the spot. This is usually followed up with an individually signed consent form after photographing. Following these procedures, we have not had any problems. Ultimately, what one is concerned about is the subject's rights and preventing the possibility of a lawsuit. Thus, a reasonable approach that is sensitive both to the individual(s) being photographed and when using the resultant images is the most critical factor when obtaining access and consent.

Fact-Finding and Sampling

Once access and consent are obtained, the fact-finding begins. For an agency or service study, the following questions must be considered:

1. What is the philosophy?
2. What are the goals and objectives of the group?
3. What are the nature and range of services offered?
4. What is the client population?
5. Who are the personnel?
6. What are the sociocultural and economic factors concerning services? Clients?
7. What are the legal implications?

Agency Survey

Once these preliminary stages of research are completed, a systematic protocol for sampling the service can be developed. The photograph represents fragmentary slices of time, so all the cautions of sampling must be respected. In agency surveys, peak leisure and midpoint activities that visually communicate segments of the service rendered should be sampled. Useful headings for the protocol include time, activity, and days. For example, in a study on adult day care, in order to better understand how a day care center functions as a care facility, we needed to know how activities varied and how they were repeated during the day's care. What times did they occur? What was the span of activities? What kinds of personnel were involved and what kinds of services were being delivered?

In a survey, the researcher is looking at a superstructure in which services are being given. The focus, then, tends to be the service as opposed to the individual. This can be difficult, as there are no individual stories told with the kind of depth which provides the cohesion that is characteristic of case studies.

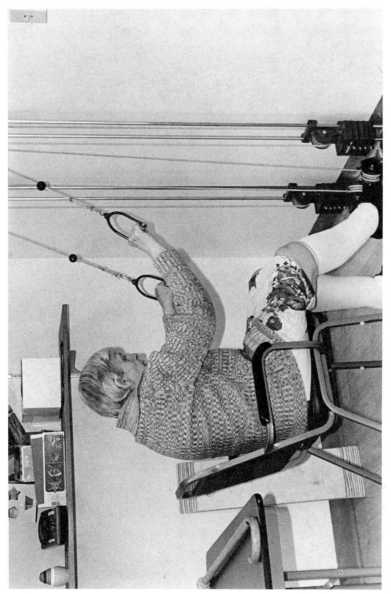

Physical therapy at San Francisco Home Health. *(Photo by Betty Highley)*

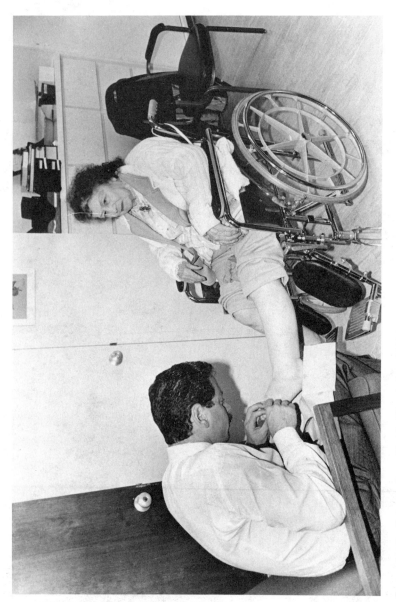

Foot care at San Francisco Home Health. (*Photo by Betty Highley*)

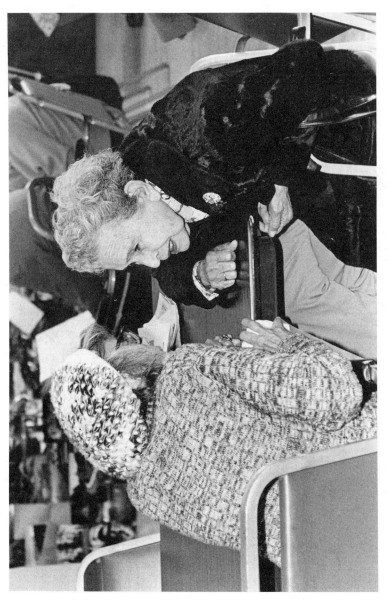

Socialization at San Francisco Home Health. (*Photo by Betty Highley*)

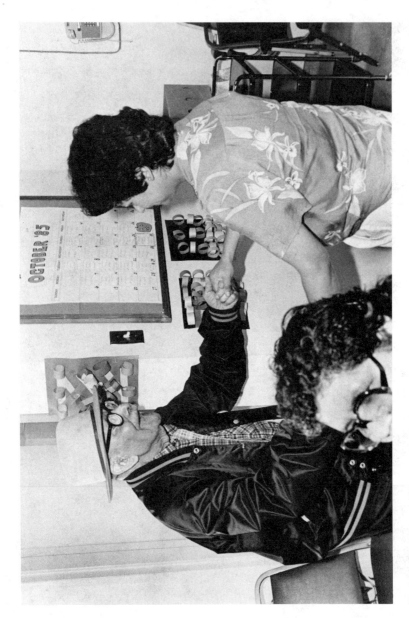

San Francisco Home Health. (*Photo by Betty Highley*)

Case Studies

The case study approach involves the examination of one situation over an extended period of time. In a study of home care of chronic illness, data is collected through photographs and interviews of patients, their family support groups, and the providers of their home care services. The purpose of the case study is to document a variety of activities so that the final combination of images presents what life is like for the study group. Photographs must be taken over a number of visits and must include a range of subjects, such as time when care is given to leisure time. The span of time covered by the photographs is often a significant factor, particularly when photographing changing conditions in long-term chronic illness; for example, where changes might not occur week to week but rather month to month or over even longer periods.

In the case study, the researcher must determine what to photograph based on a knowledge of the condition, the variables operating, and the purposes guiding the study. This requires planning and a certain amount of intuition. Interviews and conversation help identify what is pertinent to document. However, many of the most successful case studies are those in which the subjects of the study are also participants. In the final analysis, a documentary study is a collaboration between the photographer/researcher and the study subject. When this collaborative state is achieved, the documentary process can have a beneficial, therapeutic effect and the potential for a very rich study.

In a study of a home care patient with Amyotrophic Lateral Sclersosis (ALS), photographs were taken of his treatment and visits by the nurse and doctor. A trip to the hospital, which revealed the complicated mechanisms that his friends, who were his caretakers, had to go through to get him there, was also photographed. In fact, what became evident in this project was the importance of the primary caretaker, a woman who had made a major personal commitment to providing his care.

It became clear that the caretaker was of the utmost importance to the study and we wanted to investigate what she considered significant content. To do this, we left an automatic camera and some film with her for several weeks. She photographed going to the grocery store and the dentist with him in a wheelchair with a portable respirator. Her images revealed much about the social and physical obstacles they faced in the home care of this disease. Her portraits of him told much about her own feelings through how she photographed him and what else she included in the frame.

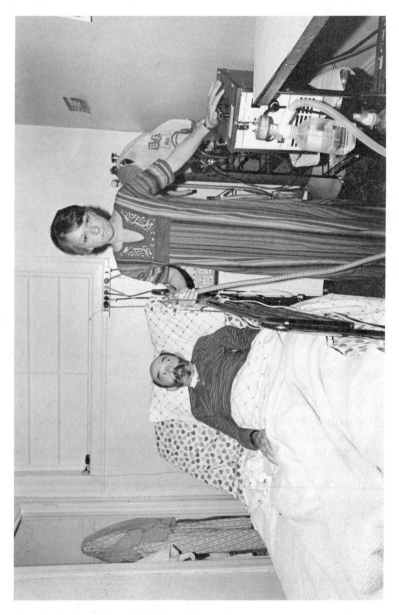

Gina trained for three months at Pacific Presbyterian Medical Center to learn to use respirators in order to care for Bill in his home. (*Photo by Tom Ferentz*)

Because the case study covers a long period of time, the final visual statement can be valuable in terms of understanding and documenting the long-term effects of care upon individuals. As a fair amount of thematic repetition exists (the same individuals seen in a variety of situations), case studies lend themselves well to public communications outside strictly academic journals and settings. Case studies can also be components of larger survey projects, in which a number of case studies are combined to offer an in-depth view of certain aspects of an agency or service.

Scripting

Scripting is another methodological design issue that relates to any photographic project. When research evolves from a knowledge base, often it is possible to chart out a project in advance. This can be an outline based on scheduled activities which direct the path of photography through an organization. In some cases, it can be extremely defined, and scripting can lead to a "shot list" or a list of photographs to be taken that show a particular care situation or variety of care. Of course, such a list is based on advance knowledge of the situation or the kind of care. One cautionary note presides, however: It is possible for the script to supersede observation with the camera at the setting, which can work against, as well as for, the investigatory nature of research. Nonetheless, scripting can be a very useful part of the design when more then one photographer is involved in recording visual data.

For example, in a study of the nutritional and food services of a home health service, knowledge about the service and clientele contributed to the development of a script. Both of the authors worked on this piece of the study. The script included such activities as the transportation service (which brought clients to the center for meals as well as delivered meals to the homes), the personnel who prepared the food and served it in the dining room, and the nutrition education program.

Analysis and Function of Photographs

How one utilizes photographs must reflect back on the original problem and purpose. The classic form of content analysis structured by procedures in documentary photography has worked best for us. We view all of the images taken at a site as a visual diary or a raw data bank. These serve as a source for analysis and are edited much like tape recordings. Although standard units of analysis—patterns, themes, numbers of people, time or space—may be used, we find that in documentary work

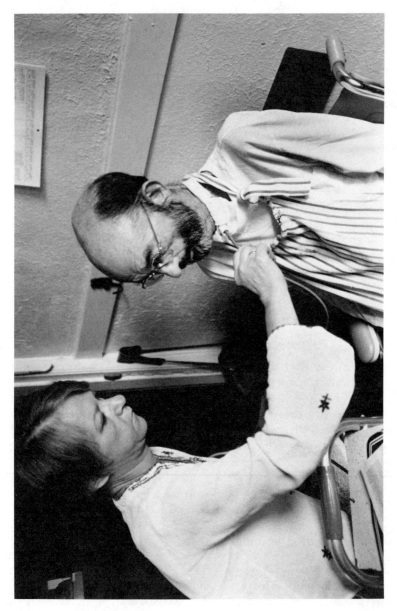

Having ALS meant that Bill had to be suctioned regularly. Gina had to be attentive to this at all times. (*Photo by Tom Ferentz*)

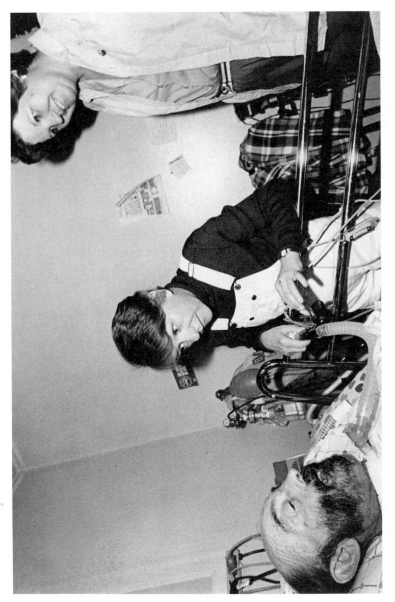

During a visit with the nurse from Visiting Nurse Association. (*Photo by Tom Ferentz*)

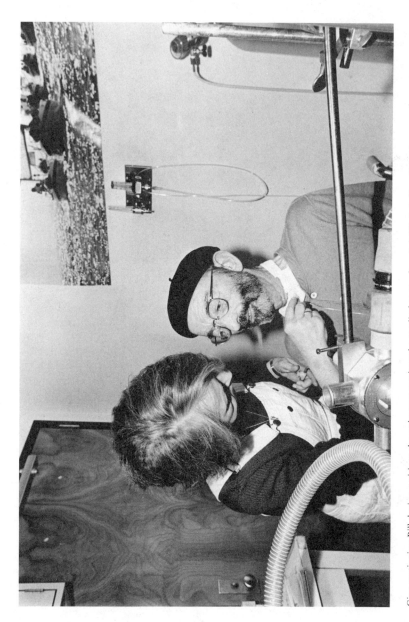

Gina suctioning Bill during a visit to the pulmonary unit at the medical center hospital. (*Photo by Tom Ferentz*)

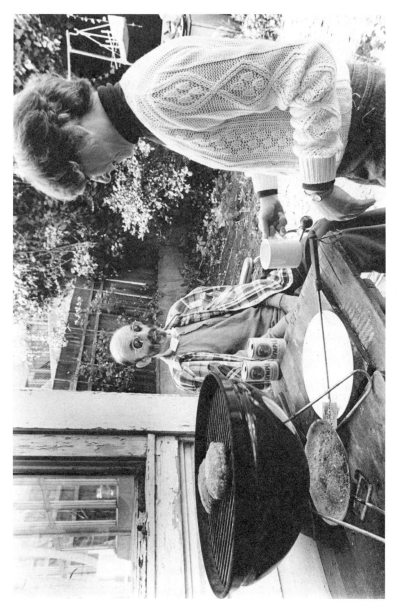

Being at home enabled Bill to participate in normal activities. (*Photo by Tom Ferentz*)

it is more often themes and patterns that we search for to provide more significant data. Once the themes are identified, we look for images that form the clearest visual statement.

Images recorded for purposes of practice and research rarely stand alone. Thus, in presentations, it is necessary to collate sequences of images that convey the dimensions of what was researched.

By freezing images and interactions on film, the photograph challenges us to find a language appropriately descriptive of the visual data. As visual evidence of what was occurring at a specific time, photographs also help us to recall details and interactions that stimulate our ability to remember while guiding it away from overly interpretive recollections. Photographs can help to stimulate and objectify the processes of memory.

The first level of analysis is done on a contact sheet (a print of all 36 exposures on a roll of film on one piece of paper). This is the raw data, and for some applications it is all that is needed. When images are used only as a visual diary, the contact sheet is adequate.

The next level of analysis is selecting patterns and themes from the contact sheet. These are made into 5 x 7 working proof prints used for further editing and analysis of content. This step is necessary when sharing the data with others, since contact sheets are difficult for more then one person to look at at a time, and they do not facilitate editing.

If the final presentation is an exhibit, book, or other publication, a final high-quality print is needed. Images selected for final prints meet more rigid criteria of content and esthetics, with emphasis placed on how they will fit into the larger context of a presentable series.

In this final stage, selected images are combined in a sequence that conveys the message or messages of the research. As the sequencing evolves, it is often necessary to return to the files or proof sheets to find images that enhance an idea that has surfaced in the work. Here is also the point at which the demand for content may sublimate the desire for esthetic standards, which is a characteristic of research and study photography that would be avoided in other areas of "artistic" photography. Naturally, it is desirable to compromise esthetics as little as possible, as they are not separable from content when "reading" photographs. Compositional design, lighting, and other formal qualities of each image express a certain synchronicity, lending themselves to greater clarity of reading. Lack of concern in this area will prove detrimental to researchers.

Finally, it is important to make as high a quality of photographic prints as possible when using them for any kind of presentation.

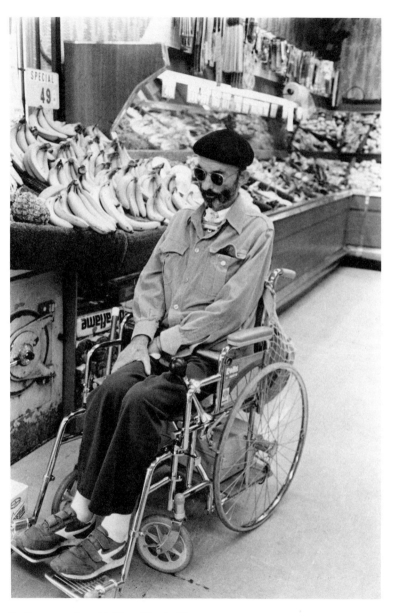

At the supermarket with Gina. (*Photo by Gina*)

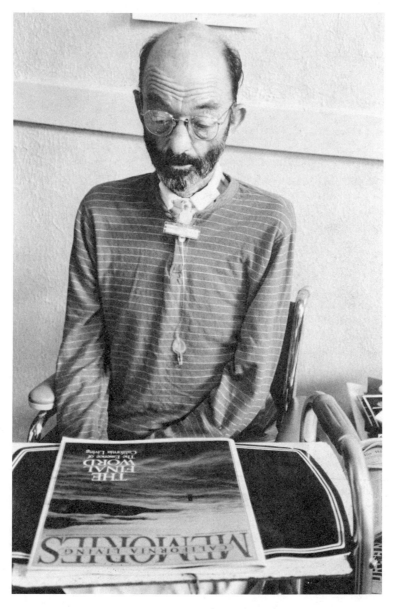

(*Photo by Gina*)

THE USES OF PHOTOGRAPHIC NURSING RESEARCH

1. *Learning more about ourselves and our work:* This reflects the most consistent commentaries from students' course evaluations in our program.

2. *Sharpening visual senses:* Students consistently say they see more and can articulate more of what they see. The need to be consistently attentive to numerous details in daily life, particularly when working in technologically complex environments, such as intensive care units, makes the ability to freeze images and study them a luxury that is often a revelation. It can attune the individual to visual data they unconsciously process but are unaware of, data that are important to them and their work. Sometimes, the act of photographing alone can do this.

3. *Communicating and educating:* Although this is a function to which much of photography applies, it specifically refers to the continuum from images as illustration in a text, to slides used in services or in a class, or to displays and exhibits.

4. *Evaluating services:* Are we really doing what we say we are doing? In our experience, photographs have revealed inconsistencies in this respect. They have shown contradictions in policy which may range from structure and organization of the physical environment to staff interactions. Because they are detailed recordings, they can be helpful in fine-tuning an agency and have even been implemental in making changes.

5. *Generating new insights and understandings:* Visual data collection is an investigative process that focuses attention on what is visible, and what is significant in the visual realm. This activity, and the subsequent analysis of still images, remains vital as a process of *discovery*.

6. *Restructuring clinical interactions:* When one begins to talk about a photo, the picture will usually stimulate a wealth of information that goes far beyond the frame of the photograph itself. This is a function most of us identify with snapshots in a family album. It is a reason that visual recording should be considered for many kinds of work and research, even when photographs are not needed in the final product.

7. *Photo interviewing:* This function has many ramifications that range from a personalized one-on-one use of images to jog the memory, to having subjects take their own pictures and interviewing them on the meaning the picture has for them. There is a great potential

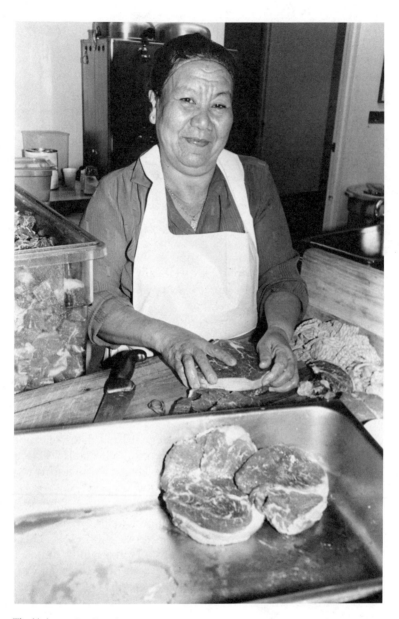

The kitchen at San Francisco Home Health. (*Photo by Betty Highley*)

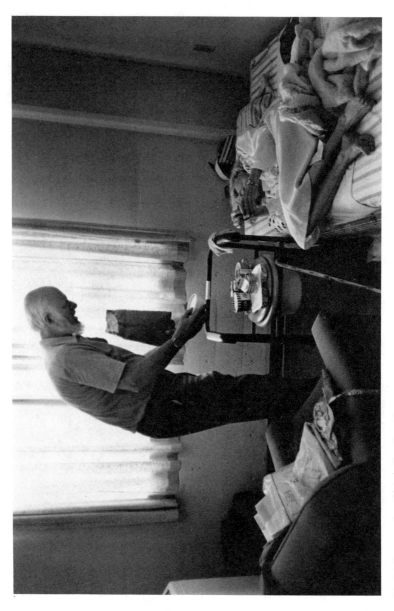

Meal delivery service. *(Photo by Tom Ferentz)*

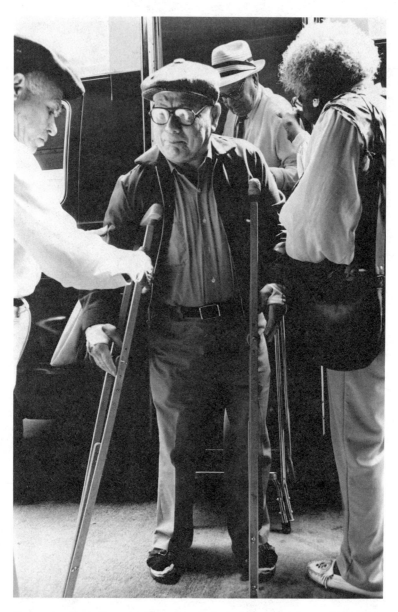

Transport service to the center for meals and other activities is a vital part of San Francisco Home Health programs. (*Photo by Betty Highley*)

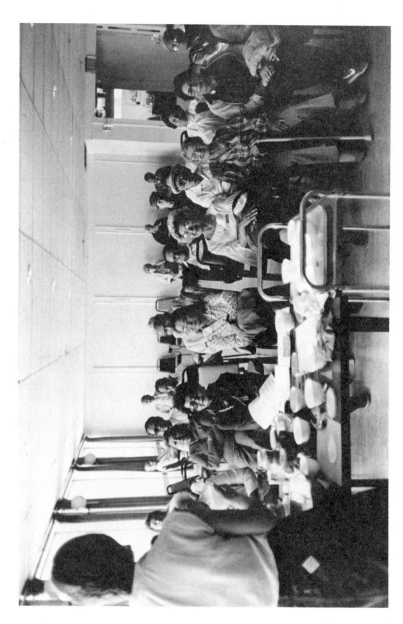

Nutrition class at San Francisco Home Health. (*Photo by Tom Ferentz*)

for interviewing with photographs that is largely untapped (Collier, 1986).

CONCLUSION

In our work, we have attempted to uncover the potentials for visual data, yet we cannot say, by any means, that we have found a comprehensive formula for its use. We have met with much encouragement from colleagues, both in nursing and in photography. At the same time, we have encountered skepticism from academics that we are playing with toys. Conversely, we have encountered criticism from photographers that we are sacrificing esthetics for content. We have little doubt that the kinds of responses we have received are similar to those experienced by visual researchers in other fields, where the methods for synthesis and analysis are not evolved enough, or not "hard" enough, or in some way do not fit in with established conventions. We feel that it is unfortunate that, with the sophistication of photography and other forms of visual media and their expansion into so many areas of the world, there is not a more established tradition in education and research emphasizing visual data.

We are pleased to have this opportunity to share some of our work and photographs. In our continued and collective search for increased understandings of unlimited and unparalleled complexities of health, illness, families, and society, we suggest that one valuable research tool is the camera.

REFERENCES

Becker, H. S. (1981). *Exploring society photographically*. Chicago: University of Chicago Press.

Capa, C. (1972). *The concerned photographer II*. New York: Grossman Publishers.

Collier, J. (1986). *Visual anthropology: Photography as a research method*. New Mexico: University of New Mexico Press.

Higgins, S. S., & Highley, B. L. (1986). The camera as a study tool: Photo interview of mothers of infants with congestive heart failure. *Children's Health Care*, *15*(2).

Johnson, W. S. (1981). *Master of photographic essay: W. Eugene Smith*. Millerton, NY: Aperture.

Lofland, J. (1971). *Analyzing social settings: A guide to qualitative observation and analysis*. Belmont, CA: Wadsworth Publishing Company, pp. 4,5, 126.

Newhall, B. (1981). *The history of photography*. New York: Museum of Modern Art.

Smith, W. E., & Smith, A. (1975). *Minimata.* New York: Holt, Rinehart, and Winston.

BIBLIOGRAPHY

Akeret, R. (1973). *Photoanalysis.* New York: Pocket Book.

Arbus, D. (1972). *Diane Arbus.* New York: Aperture Monograph.

Bellak, L., & Baker, S. (1981). *Reading faces.* New York: Holt, Rinehart and Winston.

Bellman, B. L., & Rosetto, J. (1977). *A paradigm for looking: Cross-cultural research with visual media.* Norwood, NJ: Ablex Publishing Corp.

Benner, P. (1984). *From novice to expert.* New York: Addison-Wesley.

Berger, J. (1972). *Ways of seeing.* London: British Broadcasting Co. and Penguin Books.

Berger, J. (1980). *About looking.* New York: Pantheon.

Bird, G., & Elwood, P.C. (1983). The dietary intakes of subjects estimated from photographs compared with a weighed record. *Human Nutrition: Applied Nutrition, 37A,* 470–473.

Callahan, S. (Ed.). (1972). *The photographs of Margaret Bourke-White.* New York: New York Graphic Society.

Cook, T., & Reichardt, C. (1979). *Qualitative and quantitative methods in evaluation research.* Beverly Hills: Sage Publications.

Cunningham, I. (1977). *After ninety.* Seattle: University of Washington Press.

Curtis, E. (1972). *In a sacred manner we live.* New York: Weathervane Books.

Elwood, P.C., & Bird, G. (1983) A photographic method of diet evaluation. *Human Nutrition: Applied Nutrition, 37A,* 474–477.

The encyclopedia of photography. (1970). New York: Greystone Press.

Featherstone, D. (1984). *Observations.* Carmel, CA: The friends of Photography.

Grunsky, O., & Bonacich, P. (1984). Physical contact in the family. *Journal of Marriage and the Family, 46*(3).

Hattersley, R. (1971). *Discover yourself through photography.* Dobbs Ferry, NY: Morgan & Morgan.

Heyman, T. T. (1978). *Celebrating a collection: The work of Dorothea Lange.* Oakland, CA: The Oakland Museum.

Highley, B. (1967). *Maternal role identity, defining clinical content: Graduate nursing program in maternal and child nursing.* Boulder, CO: Western Interstate Commission on Higher Education.

Higgins, S., & Highley, B. (1986, Fall). The camera as a tool: Photo interview of mothers of infants with congestive heart failure. *Children's Health Care,* 119–122.

Hirsch, J. (1981). *Family photographs: Content, meaning and effect.* New York: Oxford Press.

Julius, F. (1970). *Body language*. New York: Pocket Books.

Jussim, E. (1970). *Visual communication and the graphic arts*. New York: R.R. Bowker Co.

Kalisch, P., & Kalisch, B. (1981). When nurses were national heroines: Images of nurses in American film. *Nursing Forum, 20*(1): 14–61.

Krippendorff, K. (1980). *Content analysis: An introduction to its methodology*. Beverly Hills: Sage Publications.

Lange, D. (1967). *The American country women*. Fort Worth, TX: The Amon Carter Museum of Western Art.

Lesy, M. (1980). *Time frames: The meaning of family pictures*. New York: Pantheon Books.

Life Library of Photography. (1972). *Documentary photography*. New York: Time-Life Books.

Mark, M. E. (1981). *Falkland road*. New York: Alfred Knopf.

Masayesva, V., & Younger, E. (Eds.). *Hopi photographers Hopi images*. Tucson, AZ: Sun Tracks, University of Arizona Press.

Mead, M., & Bateson, G. (1942). *Balinese character: A photographic analysis*. New York: New York Academy of Sciences.

Mead, M. & Heyman, K. (1965). *Family*. New York: Macmillan.

Merton, T. (1956). *Silence in heaven*. New York: Studio Publications.

Newhall, B. (1980). *Photography: Essays and images*. New York: New York Graphic Society.

Newhall, B. (1982). *The history of photography*. New York: Museum of Modern Art.

Owens, B. (1973). *Suburbia*. San Francisco: Straight Arrow Books.

Owens, B. (1978). *Documentary photography: A personal view*. New York: Addison House.

Rothstein, A. (1986). *Documentary photography*. Focal Press, 1986.

Rosenberg, M. (1980). *Patients: The experience of illness*. Philadelphia: W.B. Saunders.

Ruesch, J., & Kees, W. *Nonverbal communication*. Berkeley: University of California Press.

Sedgwick, R. (1978). Photostudy as a diagnostic tool in working with families. *Current Perspectives in Psychiatric Nursing*, 60–69.

Simpson, J. (1976). *The American family: A history in photographs*. New York: Viking Press.

Smith, E. W., & Smith, A. (1972). *Master of the photographic essay*. New York: Aperture.

Sontag, S. (1977). *On photography*. New York: Dell Publishing Co.

Steichen, E. (1955). *The family of man*. New York: Museum of Modern Art.

Sussman, A. (1973). *The amateur photographer's handbook*. New York: Thomas Crowell.

Upton, B., & Upton, J. (1981). *Photography*. Boston: Little, Brown and Company.

Wagner, J. (1979). *Images of information*. Beverly Hills: Sage Publications.

Walker, E. (1971). *Walker Evans*. New York: New York Graphic Society.

Woychik, J. P., & Brickell, C. (1983, July/August). The instant camera as a therapy tool. *Social Work*, 316–318.

Zakia, R. (1979). *Perception and photography*. Rochester, NY: Light Impressions.

Zakia, R. (1980). *Perceptual quotes for photographers*. Rochester, NY: Light Impressions.

Part 4
The Ethical Path
to Nursing Knowledge

A dramatic increase in the number of scholarly investigations of ethical problems in nursing has occurred in the last five years. The issues range from metaethical questions such as "is nursing a moral activity" to the development of specific policy statements on, for example, the legalization of euthanasia or the refusal of care to patients with HIV infections. Of particular interest is the movement of some nurse ethicists away from a medical or bioethical orientation toward the development of a unique body of nursing ethics. Another trend in nursing ethical inquiry is toward a focus on micro-issues such as power and empowerment in the nurse/patient relationship and "ethical decisions at the bedside." Moral decision making in nursing is another area of active clinical investigation. The arena for ethical inquiry in nursing is vast and of utmost importance to the continuing development of the discipline.

Ethical Inquiry

Marsha Fowler and Sara Fry

ETHICAL INQUIRY

Moral knowledge, because it arises, at least in part, from a common social base, is accessible to all, even to the very young. Expressed through rules, standards, expectations and prohibitions, morality tells us to help others, to keep promises, not to steal, cheat or lie, and to be good persons. Ethics, however, is something else and aspires to something more. As a specialized field of endeavor, it is seen by ethicists as a division either of philosophy or theology. According to Frankena (1973), ethics is "philosophical thinking about morality, moral problems, and moral judgments" (p. 4). There is no doubt that ethics is also critical to the life and advancement of the profession, for ethical inquiry explores the nature of moral and ethical obligations in nursing, its standards of right conduct, and the specification of licit goods or ends to be sought by the profession as a whole or by its practitioners in the clinical setting. In this sense, it is ethics and ethical inquiry that must support and structure scientific inquiry in nursing.

MORALITY AND ETHICS: WHAT IS ETHICS?

Ethics deals with what "ought" to be, and the ways in which we discuss or think about that ought. Though it is common to use the terms *ethics* and *morality* interchangeably, there is a distinction between the two. For example, morality exists at the level of social convention, codes of behavior, general standards and rules of conduct, and community expectation. It tells us that certain kinds of actions (like lying), or that specific actions (like falsifying patient records), are either right or wrong. It also tells us whether the consequences of an action, or the motives or character traits of an individual, are good or bad. Morality refers to the additional personal rules or standards, within conventional morality, that guide the individual as well (Fowler, 1987).

On the other hand, in common discussion, the term *ethics* can have several meanings (Fry, 1986a, 1986b). For example, ethics is sometimes used to refer to the practices, beliefs, or values of a particular group of individuals, as in Christian or Jewish ethics. Ethics is also used to refer to professional ethics as described in codes of professional conduct. The American Nurses' Association (ANA) *Code for Nurses* (1976, 1985) is one document that nurses interpret as a code of professional ethics. However, in this work, the term *ethics* will mean more than beliefs or professional ethics. Specifically, it will refer to philosophical inquiry into the principles of morality (Fry, 1986a).

Ethics, as opposed to morality, is a broader, over-arching, more systematic and reflective undertaking. When an individual distances him or herself from the traditional rules of the social group, and begins to reflect upon those rules, ethical thinking has begun. A central aim of ethical thinking, for an individual, group, profession, or even a nation (Fowler, 1987), is to shape a critical and reflective morality. Ethics, then is a mode of inquiry that helps us to understand the moral dimensions of human conduct. To engage in or to *do* ethics is to undertake a particular *method* of investigation (Fry, 1986a).

THE DISCIPLINE OF ETHICS

Methods of Argumentation

Ethicists use various methods of argumentation to investigate morality (Ladd, 1978). First, there is the "appeal to authority." This appeal certifies that one ought or ought not to do some action because authority tells us to do so. The authority appealed to may be another person (i.e., mother, father), a group of persons (i.e., the profession of nursing), an institution (i.e., a church or a government), or even a hypothetical person (i.e., society). It relies on individual belief and faith in the authority appealed to.

Second, there is the "appeal to consensus" (Ladd, 1978). This appeal cites the supposed agreement of people (or groups of people) on an issue to establish its particular ethical position. Like the first method, it also relies on individual belief and faith in the people (or groups of people) who agree on the issue.

Third, there is the "appeal to intuition" (Ladd, 1978), which has a long tradition in ethics. This appeal certifies a form of ethical knowledge (self-evidence) that is often hard to refute. Like the previous methods, however, it has strength only with persons who rely on ethical intuitions. As a reliable method of ethics, it is problematic in that individual intuitions often change, over time, given a change in circumstances or the conditions that gave rise to the intuition.

Fourth and last, there is the "dialectic" or "Socratic" method (Ladd, 1978). This method asks questions and provides answers that are supported by substantial reasons and logical arguments. It also enjoys a long and respected tradition in ethics, appealing to "reason" or "rationality" for the strength of its arguments.

It is important to understand the methods of argumentation used in making ethical judgments. Of course, any ethical judgment must be supported by sound argument. Since ethical judgments often serve as a basis or rationale for moral human action, one must make sure that the method of argumentation used to reach a judgment is ethically valid and internally consistent. This is especially important since there are different subject matters in ethics.

The Subject Matter of Ethics

Ethics has several subject matters: *descriptive ethics, normative ethics, and metaethics* (Frankena, 1973). Descriptive ethics allows ethicists to inquire about the phenomena of morality and then describe and explain the phenomena in order to construct a theory of human nature that responds to ethical questions (Fry, 1986a, 1986b). Descriptive ethics also represents the work of sociologists, anthropologists, psychologists, historians, and others who describe or attempt to explain moral behavior or ends (Frankena, 1973; Beauchamp, 1983). The scientific study of moral behavior is not the same as the philosophical study of moral behavior, however, and the two should not be confused. The former seeks to answer questions such as "What does X group of people believe is right and good?" or "Why do these people behave, morally, as they do?" Nurses who scientifically study moral behavior most frequently study the values of individuals or groups (Bloomquist, Cruise, & Cruise, 1980), their levels of moral judgment (Crisham, 1981; Ketefian, 1981), or their perceptions of moral conflict (Davis, 1981) rather than inquiring into their normative and metaethical aspects.

Kohlberg's (1981) levels of moral reasoning is one type of descriptive ethical theory that is often cited by those who study moral decision making among nurses. This theory is based on studies of male children who were asked to make choices related to justice and fairness. More recent studies by Gilligan (1982), Pinch (1981), and Omery (1983), question the appropriateness of Kohlberg's theory for moral decision making in female-dominated professions, such as nursing. As a result, descriptive study of moral decision making by nurses is at a very early stage of development (Fry, 1986a, 1986b) and remains prefatory, at best.

Philosophical inquiry related to the standards or criteria of right or wrong conduct, and moral action, in general, is usually contained within *normative ethics*. It begins with the question, "What ought I to do?" From this vantage, the ethicist then examines various principles, rules, or standards of right or wrong commonly appealed to for moral conduct. It also allows the ethicist to assess the moral weight of our perceived duties and obligations in human interaction and propose ethical theories for moral human conduct using the various methods of argumentation to assert the worth of these theories (Fry, 1986a).

Normative ethics allows the ethicist to ask questions about specific principles, such as "What is a just allocation of social resources?" or "What characteristics does a 'good' person possess?" Employing this method, the ethicist focuses on evaluative judgments in an attempt to identify moral obligations, duties, and values that ought to guide individual or group moral action. Because it leads to applied ethics, normative ethics is that division of ethics most practicing health professionals are concerned about (Fowler, 1987) (see Figure 1).

Figure 1
Ethics as a Discipline: Its Divisions

Non-Normative Ethics		**Normative Ethics**
Descriptive Ethics	Metaethics	General Normative Ethics
The scientific, non-philosophical, study of ethics. Provides a factual description of moral behavior and belief systems or beliefs.	Analysis of meaning, justification, and inferences of moral terms, concepts, and statements.	Formulation and defense of basic principles, values, virtues and ideals governing moral behavior. (See Figure 2 for division of normative ethics.)

Adapted from Fowler (1984).

Within normative ethics, there are two major divisions. The first deals with decisions about what is *right* or *wrong to do*. Such judgments are called *norms of obligation* because they tell us what our moral obligations and duties are.

Normative ethics also tells us what is *good* and *evil* or *good* and *bad* in persons, groups, motives or things. Judgments of what is good or evil in persons are called *norms of moral value*, and attempt to resolve such questions as "what are the characteristics of a 'good' person?" Examples of moral values, known as virtues, include humility, generosity, and wisdom (Fowler, 1987).

Judgments of what is good or bad in things or ends we seek or desire are called *norms of nonmoral value*. Norms of nonmoral value allow the ethicist to answer questions that often seem of peripheral interest to ethics; for example, "what is a 'good' birthing experience?" There are hundreds of categories of nonmoral values. Some are things that "are good in themselves," or possessing intrinsic value (such as human life). Some are "instrumental" or possessing a value that allows us to reach other ends. Health, for example, can be considered instrumental in this way as it allows us to live a "life that is meaningful and manageable" (ANA, Social Policy, 1980), and to realize other important values. Although judgments of nonmoral value are in fact normative judgments, not all normative judgments are normative *ethical* judgments. Judgments of nonmoral value belong to the field of *axiology*, and are not regarded by ethicists as a part of ethics proper (Frankena, 1973). This is not to say, however, that they are not important: they are; they pertain to ethics because they influence ethical decisions and designate the goods or ends groups and individuals seek, such as health, happiness, or prosperity. (Frankena, 1973) (see Figure 2).

Metaethics, which is usually studied by professional ethicists alone, is primarily concerned with theoretical issues of meaning and justification, or logical, epistemological, and semantic questions in ethics. Metaethics addresses such questions as "Why be good?" or "Is the good good because the gods have ordained it, or do the gods ordain the good because it is good," (Plato, 1953). Metaethics also prompts the ethicist to ask such questions as "What do we mean when we say that X (a particular value or action) is 'good' or 'right' (or 'just' or any moral term)?" These more speculative sorts of questions are what people sometimes think of as ethics. Such questions often are wrongly viewed as impractical theorizing. However, though their practical import may not be immediately visible, they are critical to the work of ethics.

For the professional ethicist, metaethics involves a secondary level of

Figure 2
Normative Ethics

Theories of Obligation		Theories of Value	
Deontological Theories	Teleological Theories	Moral Value	Nonmoral Value
A given action is right or wrong based upon an intrinsic quality, its conformity with a moral rule, or factors other than the consequences produced.	An action is right or wrong insofar as it produces a particular nonmoral good/ value or produces a greater amount or balance of that good than could any alternative action.	Analysis of what is virtuous or evil in persons.	Analysis of what is good or bad in things or ends that are sought.

Applied Normative Ethics	Moral Policy Formulation
Application and interaction of general normative ethics to specific issues, cases or problems within a discipline or profession; includes bioethics, business ethics, legal ethics, etc.	An aspect of applied normative ethics. Includes the formulation of broad guides which incorporate moral norms of a social or professional group, which have ramifications outside the group, reflect the value perspective of the group, and speak to issues requiring social change or professional consistency. Moral policy formulation involves group decision making and activity and the expenditure or allocation of resources to achieve policy ends.

Adapted from D. Fowler (1984).

philosophical inquiry into the nature of ethical inquiry itself. For the professional ethicist, such inquiry promotes theories *about* ethics, rather than theories *for* ethical conduct. Metaethics, therefore, allows ethicists to investigate the relationships between human conduct and morality, between ethical beliefs (values) and the facts of the real world, as well as the relationships among ethical theories, principles, rules, and human conduct (Veatch & Fry, 1987).

In summary, the various subject matters of ethics are related in significant ways. For example, we would engage in descriptive ethics to describe moral phenomena (such as the duty to protect patients from harm) within health care practices. We would then engage in normative ethics in order to argue a specific principle or rule in a particular case situation. Last, we would engage in metaethics to inquire about the nature of that moral principle in nursing, or to inquire *about* normative ethics.

NORMS OF OBLIGATION

Ethicists distinguish ethical theories from one another by the various methods employed to determine what is right or wrong. Teleological and deontological ethics, the two major theories that specify norms of obligation, are discussed below.

Teleological Ethics

Teleological ethics, (from *telos*, Greek for *end*) allows the ethicist to determine an action to be right or wrong based on the consequences the action produces. Teleological ethics are sometimes called consequentialistic ethics. For example, because hedonism and stoicism determine the rightness or wrongness of an action based upon the consequences produced, both fall within the category of teleological theories. In consequentialistic ethics, however, it is more than consequences alone that the ethicist examines. An action is right or wrong based upon the consequences produced, *as measured over against a specific end that is sought, a nonmoral value*, such as pleasure, or dispassion, or utility. This is precisely the point at which norms of nonmoral value become important to ethics. It is nonmoral values, such as pleasure, which are the *telos*, the ends, of teleological theories. Stated another way, in teleological ethics, that which is right (to do) is a function of that which is good (to seek or cherish) and is expressed as such in teleological theories. Here, obligations are inextricably tied to nonmoral values (Fowler, 1987).

Utilitarian Ethics.   *Utilitarian ethics* remains the most important teleological theory for contemporary health care. Founded by theologian John Gay in England during the 1700s, Utilitarianism was subsequently developed by Jeremy Bentham, James Mill, John Stuart Mill, Henry Sigwick, Hastings Rashdall, and G.E. Moore, among others.

In effect, Utilitarianism asserts that a right act is one that produces the greatest amount of pleasure or happiness over pain. For this, there must be some method by which pleasure can be evaluated; Bentham, for example, created a "calculus" by which pleasure could be "measured." The calculus includes an assessment of the intensity, duration, certainty/ uncertainty, propinquity, fecundity, and purity of the pleasure (in Melden, 1967). Pleasure, then, according to Bentham, was to be understood in terms of utility, and especially social utility.

Soon after, J. S. Mill modified and enhanced Bentham's Utilitarianism by proposing the principle of the "greatest good for the greatest number." Although this principle, as stated here, remains a popular understanding of Mill, it does disservice to his work by oversimplifying it. Mill's Utilitarianism is better understood as seeking "the greatest possible balance of value over disvalue for all persons who would be affected" (Mill, 1957). That is, while Utilitarian theories can judge the rightness or wrongness of an action on a situation-by-situation basis, Mill and subsequent Utilitarians leaned toward a form of Utilitarianism based on an overriding premise: that *adherence to certain moral rules* will generally produce the greatest value over disvalue in their consequences. For example, rather than judging the utility of single acts, situationally (referred to as Act Utilitarianism), Mill and others have preferred to judge utility through the use of rules (called Rule Utilitarianism) (Fowler, 1987).

However, there are ethical theories that depend upon some aspect other than consequences to determine the rightness or wrongness of an action. These theories do not maintain that consequences are unimportant, only that they are not constitutive of the right. These theories are usually termed *deontological* (from *deon*, Greek for *duty*) or *formalist* theories. The German philosopher Immanuel Kant is the chief representative of ethical formalism.

Deontological Ethics

In deontological ethics, the intrinsic quality of the action itself or its conformity to a rule, determines the rightness or wrongness of the action, irrespective of consequences. For instance, breaking a promise could be considered to be intrinsically wrong. Most situations, however, have extenuating circumstances; in some instances, it would be better to break than to keep a specific promise, particularly if the promise was trivial, and breaking it could save a life.

Ethical formalism generally results in the use of principles or their derivative rules to guide decision making. Keeping promises, telling the truth, and not disclosing private information are examples of such rules. In view of the fact that rules can produce untoward results when kept absolutely, perhaps it is better stated that promise keeping is "right making," if not always right. In ethical formalism, rules are regarded as *contentless forms* (hence the term formalism). Forms are rules without specification, without content. For example, "thou shalt not kill," is a contentless form. It does not define killing, neither does it specify conditions under which killing might be socially permissible. Yet it is clear that killing is done in civilized societies (war, self-defense, capital punishment, accident, use of animals for food). It is also clear that killing must be justified, as unjustified killing is severely punished. "Thou shalt not kill" is a general rule that society upholds, but gives content when applied to specific situations. One reformulation of the rule that gives it content is this: "It is always wrong directly to take innocent human life." This restatement adds content, sufficient to permit killing in a narrow range of cases, while prohibiting others and upholding the general rule (Fowler, 1987).

Rules

What constitues a moral rule? Principles, in order to be valid rules, must meet certain conditions. Kant, in his "categorical imperative," formulated one condition, in three statements, that must be satisfied in order for a moral rule to be considered valid. Taylor (1975) provides us with a particularly understandable statement of the categorical imperative in its reformulation. It is:

1. For a rule to be a rule, it must be consistently universalizable.
2. For a rule to be a moral rule, it must be such that, if all men follow it, they would treat each other as ends in themselves, and never as means only.
3. For a rule to be a moral rule, it must be capable of being self-imposed by the will of each person when he or she is universally legislating. (p. 88)

In part, these reformulations specify that valid moral rules should be applicable to all persons, without exception; second, that rules must lead to treating the persons involved as persons of absolute worth, as ends, not merely as means to another's ends; third, that persons who choose to embrace a rule as self-chosen, and are not coerced to accept it, acknowledge the universally valid nature of that rule. These conditions give rise to the principles and rules which are often discussed in bioethical literature: principles of justice, autonomy, nonmaleficence, beneficence, fidelity, veracity, confidentiality, and so forth.

Principles and Rules.   The distinction between principles and rules is generally this: principles are basic, and rules are derived from principles. While different authors identify different principles, this does not reflect any dispute over the importance of the different principles. Rather, it reflects differences in opinion as to which are basic principles and which are derived rules. In the end, most theories, whether teleological or deontological, focus upon ethical principles and rules as action guides. Both Utilitarianism and Kantianism result in the use of principles and rules in ethical decision making. Utilitarians use rules because their use will generally produce consequences which most closely approximate the ends they seek. Deontologists use rules because they are judged to be intrinsically right-making, irrespective of the consequences they may produce in any particular situation. However, principles, as norms of obligation, must not be confused with norms of value (Fowler, 1987).

NORMS OF VALUE

Norms of Moral Value

Norms of obligation specify what our duties and obligations are. Norms of value specify what we are to be or to seek as goods or ends. Those norms of value that allow ethicists to identify what is good or bad, or virtuous and evil, in *persons* are called *norms of moral value*. Norms of moral value are also called *virtues*. According to Frankena (1973), virtues are habits of character which predispose a person to meet his or her duty, to do what is right. They are learned, practiced, and developed, not a matter of personality.

Excellences, a subset of virtue, are those habits of character which predispose a person to do a specific skill or task well (Aristotle, 1962). They are the traits of character that one would see in, for example, a "good nurse," Unfortunately, too little attention is given to identifying and fostering the excellences necessary to nursing practice.

Since the late 1950s or early 1960s, an ethics of virtue, once so prominent in nursing's ethics, has given way to emphasis on an ethics of obligation (Fowler, 1984). In the last decade, however, there has been a recrudescence of virtue theory in ethics, in part because the two approaches to ethics must go hand-in-hand. As Frankena (1973) parodies Kant, "principles without traits are impotent and traits without principles are blind" (p.65).

Norms of Nonmoral Value

Moral values pertain to persons while nonmoral values pertain to non-persons. Norms of nonmoral value, the goods and ends we seek, are intrinsic to every human endeavor, nursing included. Nursing itself cherishes values such as human dignity, well being, and human worth. Other less global values are also part of nursing: comfort, care, respect, and meaningful life. Here, documents such as the ANA's *Social Policy Statement* (1980) are particularly important to discussions of nonmoral values in the profession. Statements such as ". . . health [is] the center of nursing attention, not as an end in itself, but as a means to life that is meaningful and manageable" (p. 6) are critical to the analysis of the *telos* of nursing, as well as the goals and conduct of patient care.

PROFESSIONAL ETHICS AND POLICY FORMULATION

Normative ethics gives rise to several subdivisions of relevance to nursing practice. Norms of obligation and norms of value combine to produce two areas. First, there is the field of applied ethics and its various sub-categories. Every discipline or profession has its particular ethical concerns. Medicine has its own law, divinity its own law, business its own law, and nursing its own law. Professional ethics is one type of applied ethics. Biomedical ethics, ethics applied to the biomedical sciences, is also a form of applied ethics. Hence, both nursing and medical ethics can be viewed as subtypes of "bioethics."

Second, there is the field of moral policy formulation. Moral policy formulation involves the process of giving voice, through policies and position statements, to professional obligations and values in terms of their contact with specific societal issues.

What is Biomedical Ethics?

During the last 25 years, the tremendous growth of knowledge and rapid technological advancements have created unprecedented moral questions. "Ought I to keep this patient alive?" for example, was a moral question that simply did not arise when there was no capability of sustaining life with artificial life-support mechanisms. However, once increased knowledge and technology made it possible to affect human existence by dramatically altering life, death, and how we experience life, such "ought" questions arose by the score to force new types of moral decisions. According to Clouser (1978), such questions also created a new mode of inquiry within ethics: biomedical ethics or applied ethics in the biomedical sciences.

For example, the fundamental and traditional moral injunction against killing others created difficult decisions for health professionals when it became evident that turning off life-support systems directly "caused" death. These decisions were doubly difficult when the patient was suffering a slow, debilitating death or was in intractable pain. When forced to choose between sustaining an undignified human existence and terminating life, many health professionals faced severe moral conflict. This type of conflict is the classic example of the moral dilemma where opposing actions exist, each of which can be ethically justifiable (Beauchamp & Childress, 1983). To not disconnect life-sustaining machinery in such situations is to sustain life and avoid killing, a preeminent duty of the health professional. To disconnect the equipment is to respect human dignity and avoid pain, also a preeminent duty of the health professional. Although directly conflictive, each action can be justified by traditional moral principles (Fry, 1986a).

To respond to the particular nature of these types of decisions, health professionals found that their codes of ethics were of insufficient assistance. In order to decide, "What ought I to do?" health professionals looked toward traditional ethics for moral theories and methods of argumentation that could be applied to the biomedical sciences. The development of biomedical ethics (sometimes referred to as "bioethics"), as a field of ethical inquiry, emerged and subsequently evolved through several stages (Walters, 1978).

The first, and most general, stage was medical ethics, which included philosophical inquiry into the ethical norms for the conduct of medicine (Veatch, 1981). The development of professional codes of medical ethics, the Hippocratic tradition, and the influences of secular/non-secular ethical traditions on medical ethics express central themes of concern here. Scholars of medical ethics early on claimed that all applications of ethics to problems in the medical sphere are part of medical ethics (Veatch, 1981). Physician ethics, nursing ethics, social work ethics, dentist ethics, and chaplain ethics were offered by scholars as examples of the various branches of medical ethics. However, recent works in some areas of clinical practice seem to indicate that a few practices view themselves as substantially different from medical ethics and from each other (Fowler,

1984; Jameton, 1984; Reamer, 1982). A rapidly growing area of ethical discourse, business ethics, is also an area of professional ethics that does not fit the early descriptions of professional ethics in clinical practices (Hoffman & Moore, 1984). To delineate some of its differences, nursing is beginning to engage in descriptive ethics in order to clearly depict the moral phenomena of nursing that are distinct from the moral phenomena of other clinical practices (Ketefian, 1985). All of these efforts are enlarging our understanding of the application of biomedical ethics to health care and professional practices.

The second stage of development in biomedical ethics has occurred along with attempts to gain new knowledge through systematic human experimentation (Walters, 1978). Codes of research ethics (protection of human subjects in research), and the social and moral consequences of research and new technologies (cost/benefit analyses; technology assessment of the artificial heart, for example) exemplify central themes of this stage.

The third stage of development in biomedical ethics has evolved with the effort to formulate public policy guidelines for clinical care, biomedical research, and the allocation of health care resources (Walters, 1978). Legislated committees and groups to study these problems and to formulate recommendations for public policy on these matters have included the National Commission for the Protection of Human Subjects of Biomedical and Behavioral Research (National Research Act, 1974), the Ethics Advisory Board Report (1979), and the President's Commission for the Study of Ethical Problems in Medicine and Biomedical Research (1982). The President's Commission was particularly productive in issuing public reports and recommendations on a variety of ethical issues of interest to nurses and others engaged in clinical practices.

In each stage of its development, biomedical ethics has used the traditional subject areas of ethics and appealed to traditional methods in applying ethical reasoning to biomedical contexts. It is an important and widely accepted field of inquiry in ethics that is just beginning to be utilized and developed within the discipline of nursing (Fry, 1986a).

Why is Biomedical Ethics Important to Nursing Practice?

To understand why biomedical ethics is important to nursing practice, one must consider the underlying moral foundations of nursing practice and the manner in which nursing has articulated them. In the preamble to the ANA *Code for Nurses* (1985), it is stated that the most fundamental principle underlying nurses' clinical judgments is the principle of *respect for persons.* Other principles are derived from this basic principle and function as action guides for nursing judgments and actions, including: autonomy (self-determination), beneficence (doing good), nonmalefi-cence (avoiding harm), veracity (truth-telling), confidentiality (respecting privileged information), fidelity (keeping promises), and justice (treating people fairly). Basic understanding of these principles and their moral dimensions is a necessary first step to ethical inquiry in nursing.

Autonomy.   According to Veatch and Fry (1987), this principle claims that individuals are to be permitted personal liberty to determine their own actions according to plans they themselves have chosen. To respect persons as autonomous individuals is to acknowledge their personal choices.

Beneficence.   According to Frankena (1973), the principle of beneficence states that "we ought to do good and prevent or avoid doing harm" (p. 45). Veatch and Fry (1987) have interpreted this to mean that nurses are morally obligated to provide benefits to patients in terms of goods or assets.

Nonmaleficence.   According to Frankena (1973), this principle obliges the nurse *not* to inflict evil or harm on patients. It is the nurse's duty to protect the patient from harm.

For the nurse, this duty is derived, in part, from the profession's perceived obligation to benefit the patient and protect him or her from harm. This obligation takes on additional meaning in special relation-ships, such as the nurse–patient relationship, where the implicit contract underlying the nature of the relationship indicates that positive benefit-ing or acts of beneficence should take place. In the ANA *Code for Nurses* (1985), this obligation stresses a central ethical duty: "The nurse's primary commitment is to the client's care and safety" (p. 8). In being accountable, the nurse is directly answerable for what he or she has done in terms of this duty. To be accountable means to give good reasons—moral reasons—for the mode and manner one chooses to protect the patient from harm (Fry, 1986a). It is the central obligation in nursing and, unfortunately, the least understood.

Veracity.   According to Veatch and Fry (1987), this principle is usually defined as the obligation to tell the truth and not to lie or deceive. People have long regarded truthfulness as fundamental to the existence of trust among individuals. In health care relationships, truthfulness gains particular significance. As the interpretive statements to the ANA *Code for Nurses* (1985) point out, "Truth telling and the process of reaching informed choice underlie the exercise of self-determination, which is basic to respect for persons" (p. 2). The nurse is obliged to respect a principle of veracity in providing nursing care to patients.

Confidentiality.   According to Veatch and Fry (1987), the principle of confidentiality recognizes that maintenance of privileged information is one of the most basic ethical requirements of professional health care ethics. Although keeping confidentiality is not an absolute requirement in nursing, the expectation of confidentiality seems fundamental to the trust relationship between nurse and patient and often assumes the status of a right independent of consequences to others. According to the ANA (1985), confidentiality may be broken only when "innocent parties are in direct jeopardy" (p. 4).

Fidelity.   According to Veatch and Fry (1987), the principle of fidelity guides one in remaining faithful to one's commitments, especially to keeping promises. Individuals generally expect that promises will be kept in all human relationships. At least, promises should not be broken unless there is a good reason to break them.

One of the fundamental promises inherent in the nurse–patient relationship is the nurse's implicit promise to care for the patient. Indeed, the caring phenomenon is considered by Fry (1988) to be the central ethic in nursing, yet the extent to which nurses can keep this promise to patients is often dependent on the context of nursing care and the presence of external constraints on nursing practice. Although it is a very important moral principle in nursing practice, it is often hard to honor within the realities of the health care arena.

Justice.   The last ethical principle is that of justice or the obligation to treat people fairly. According to Veatch and Fry (1987), justice is the principle that is usually appealed to in making decisions about how benefits and burdens ought to be distributed among patients. Depending on the theory of justice that one adopts, this principle forms the basis of most resource allocation decisions in health care.

When nurses take all of the moral principles into consideration in their decision making and appeal to these principles in making normative arguments about what the nurse *ought* to do, they are engaging in ethical inquiry. To *do* ethics in nursing is to undertake a particular method of investigation, using the principles and methods of ethics, into matters of moral concern regarding patient care. In so doing, the nurse will find that these principles often will be prioritized in forming a moral judgment or in carrying out a moral action. Understanding the manner in which nurses prioritize these principles and their relative importance to one another is, therefore, also a form of ethical inquiry. Application of these principles to specific issues for the purposes of the development of position statements or guidelines is a part of moral policy formulation.

Moral Policy Formulation

Policy issues and policy formulation are crucial to ethics from at least two perspectives. First, it is through policy statements and guidelines that the norms of a group are given public voice and force. Second, there are few policy issues that do not have a moral aspect.

Sound policy formulation and enactment is critical to the practitioner. It is policy which allows the professional to act upon the ethical norms of the profession within society. Policies set forth official professional expectations and allow for the development of mechanisms and processes for relevant action. These expectations, then, become the standards of the profession by which individual professional actions are judged. Policies also serve as standards for professional groups themselves in terms of their long-range goals, the allocation of organizational resources, or the establishment of professional priorities (Fowler, 1987).

Moral policy formulation is also important to a profession in that it is one aspect of broader policy formulation processes. There are few issues in society, or within a profession, which are solely moral issues and of no interest to the law or other regulation. However, there are few significant policies which do not contain a moral element. It is ludicrous to think that a policy on the allocation of health care resources for the elderly could be free of any consideration of justice, a specifically moral concern. Likewise, "Baby Doe" and "Grandpa Doe" policies or regulations cannot be written without some regard for treatment and the moral discussion surrounding the quality/sanctity of life debate. Thus, when moral policy does not stand alone, it can be incorporated into broader policy concerns which address large social issues.

Policy and position statements are also developed by professional organizations and professional specialty groups. In late 1983 (revised 1987), the ANA published a position statement on the nurse's participation in capital punishment by lethal injection. Statements like this are generally understood to represent the position of the profession as a whole on an issue. The California Nurses' Association (1987) statement on nurse participation in active euthanasia provides another example. Other specialty organizations, such as the American Association of Critical-Care Nurses (AACN), also formulate policy and develop position statements on specific issues of social import. For example, in 1984 AACN published a statement entitled *AACN's Statement on Ethics in Critical-Care Research.*

When nurses utilize and appeal to moral principles to develop normative policies or to analyze the moral components of preexisting or proposed policies, they are engaging in a form of ethical inquiry. They are working to analyze or establish normative positions on matters of moral concern with regard to direct patient care or to broader social issues that will affect care or the moral aspects of the nurse–patient relationship.

CONCLUSION

Ethical inquiry, though it has received increased attention since the 1960s, and though it has touched upon all three stages of development of bioethics, is as yet nascent in the nursing profession. There are many questions that remain to be addressed or to be addressed more fully. These questions are both wide-ranging and foundational. Questions on the moral nature of accountability and responsibility, or advocacy, or of caring come to mind. Issues in the distinctiveness of nursing ethics over and against medical ethics require further study. Clinical concerns raise such questions as whether or not it is morally permissible for nurses to conduct nontherapeutic research on patients who cannot participate in the research process. Social issues, such as those discussed by Fowler (1984), regarding "what is the nature, role and force of compensatory justice in nursing practice?" also raise important ethical questions for nurses.

Finally, ethical inquiry itself, as an exploration of the nature of ethical obligations in nursing, its standards of right conduct, and the moral appropriateness of the goods and ends the profession and its members seek, is foundational to the development of nursing's science and practice.

REFERENCES

American Association of Critical-Care Nurses. (1984). *AACN's statement on ethics in critical-care research.* Newport Beach, CA: Author.

American Nurses' Association. (1980). *Nursing: A social policy statement.* Kansas City, MO: Author, p. 6.

American Nurses' Association. (1985). *Code for nurses with interpretive statements.* Kansas City, MO: Author.

American Nurses' Association Committee on Ethics. (1988). *Statement on nurse's participation in capital punishment.* Kansas City, MO: Author.

Aristotle. (1962). *Nichomachean ethics.* (M. Ostwald, Trans.). Indianapolis: Bobbs-Merrill, p. 33.

Beauchamp T. L., & Childress, J. F. (1983). *Principles of biomedical ethics* (2nd ed.). New York: Oxford.

Bentham, J. (1967). The principles and morals of legislation. In A.I. Melden (Ed.), *Ethical theories: A book of readings.* (2nd ed.). Englewood Cliffs, NJ: Prentice-Hall.

Bloomquist, B. L., Cruise, P. D., & Cruise, R. J. (1980). Values of baccalaureate nursing students in secular and religious schools. *Nursing Research, 29,* 379–383.

California Nurses' Association Ethics Committee. (1987). *Position statement on nurse participation in active euthanasia for the terminally ill.* San Francisco: Author.

Chrisham, P. (1981). Measuring moral judgment in nursing dilemmas. *Nursing Research. 30,* 104–110.

Clouser, K. D. (1978). In W. T. Riech (Ed.), *Encyclopedia of bioethics,* vol 1. New York: The Free Press.

Davis, A. (1981). Ethical dilemmas in nursing: A survey, *Western Journal of Nursing Research. 3*(4), 397–407.

Ethics Advisory Board. (1979). Report. *Federal Register,* 44 (No. 118) June 18, 1979, 35033-35058.

Fowler, M. D. M. (1984). *Ethics and nursing, 1893–1984: The ideal of service, the reality of history.* Unpublished manuscript.

Fowler, M. D. M. (1987). Introduction to ethics and ethical theory: A road map to the discipline. In M. D. M. Fowler & J. Levine-Ariff (Eds.), *Ethics at the bedside: A source book for the critical-care nurse.* Philadelphia: JB Lippincott.

Frankena, W. K. (1973). *Ethics.* Englewood Cliffs, NJ: Prentice-Hall.

Fry, S. T. (1986a). Ethical inquiry in nursing: The definition and method of biomedical ethics. *Perioperative Nursing Quarterly, 2,* 1–8.

Fry, S. T. (1986b). Ethical inquiry in nursing: The state of the art. *Virginia Nurse, 54,* 12–13.

Fry, S. T. (1988). The ethics of caring: Can it survive in nursing? *Nursing Outlook, 36,* 48.

Gilligan, C. (1982). *In a different voice: Psychological theory and women's development.* Cambridge: Harvard University Press.

Jameton, A. (1984). *Nursing practice: The ethical issues.* Englewood Cliffs, NJ: Prentice-Hall.

Jones, W. T. (1969). *The classical mind: A history of western philosophy.* (2nd ed.). New York: Harcourt, Brace & World.

Hoffman, W. M., & Moore, I. M. (1984). *Business ethics: Readings and cases in corporate morality.* New York: McGraw-Hill.

Kant, E. (1959). *Foundations of the metaphysics of morals* (L. Beck, Trans.). Indianapolis, IN: Bobbs-Merrill.

Ketefian, S. (1981). Critical thinking, education preparation, and development or moral judgment among selected groups of practicing nurses. *Nursing Research, 30,* 98–103.

Ketefian, S. (1985). Professional and bureaucratic role conceptions and moral behavior among nurses. *Nursing Research, 32,* 248–253.

Kohlberg, L. (1981). *The philosophy of moral development: Moral stages and the idea of justice.* San Francisco: Harper & Row.

Ladd, J. (1978). The task of ethics. In W. T. Riech (Ed.), *Encyclopedia of bioethics,* vol 1., pp. 401–407. New York: The Free Press.

Melden, A. I. (Ed.). (1976). *Ethical theories: A book of readings* (2nd ed. rev.). Englewood-Cliffs, NJ: Prentice-Hall.

Mill, J. S. (1957). *Utilitarianism.* Indianapolis: Bobbs-Merrill Educational Publishing.

National Research Act of 1974, Title III, Public Law 93–348 and 95–622.

Omery, A. (1983). Moral development: A differential evaluation of dominant models. *Advances in Nursing Science, 6,* 1–17.

Pinch, J. W. (1981). Feminine attributes in a masculine world. *Nursing Outlook, 29,* 596–599.

Plato. (1953). *Euthyphro, Apology, Crito, and Symposium.* South Bend, IN: Gateway Editions, Ltd., p. 13.

President's Commission for the Study of Ethical Problems in Medicine and Biomedical Research. (1982). *Making health care decisions.* Washington, DC: U.S. Government Printing Office.

President's Commission for the Study of Ethical Problems in Medicine and Biomedical Research. (1983). *Deciding to forego life-sustaining treatment.* Washington, DC: U.S. Government Printing Office.

President's Commission for the Study of Ethical Problems in Medicine and Biomedical Research. (1983). *Securing access to health care.* Washington, DC: U.S. Government Printing Office.

Reamer, F. G. (1982). *Ethical dilemmas in social services.* New York: Columbia University Press.

Taylor, P. (1975). *Principles of ethics: An introduction.* Belmont, CA: Dickinson.

Veatch, R. M. (1981). *A theory of medical ethics.* New York: Basic Books.

Veatch, R., & Fry, S. T. (1987). *Case studies in nursing ethics.* Philadelphia: J. B. Lippincott.

Walters, L. (1978). Bioethics as a field of ethics. In T. L. Beauchamp & L. Walters (Eds.). *Contemporary issues in bioethics.* Belmont, CA: Wadsworth.

Part 5
The Intellectual/
Interpretive Path
to Nursing Knowledge

Intellectual/interpretive modes of inquiry involve the creative use of the intellect to solve problems of significance to the discipline. Dr. Stephenie Edgerton, a professor of philosophy at New York University who has mentored an entire generation of new nurse philosophers, prepared the first chapter in this section. Dr. Edgerton has been intimately involved in the introduction of philosophical research as a powerful tool in the development of nursing knowledge. Philosophical research in nursing has, without doubt, challenged the discipline and raised its theoretical and metaparadigmatic discussions to new heights of sophistication and clarity. Also known as foundational research, it does indeed work at the very foundation of the discipline—its world view, values, goals, and perspectives. Philosophical studies in nursing have dealt with such questions as the meanings of health and holism, the nature of nursing knowledge, the existential significance of illness and suffering, the nature of human life, and the philosophical sources and implications of various nursing theories. Such issues and innumerable others demand rigorous exploration by nursing scholars.

Philosophical Analysis

Stephenie G. Edgerton

Although philosophers disagree as to what precisely constitutes philosophical analysis, it is possible to describe the philosophical tradition and its intellectual modes of inquiry. Therefore, this paper will characterize the reflective activities philosophers engage in and have engaged in since the time of the Greeks. Of special concern to nursing is the inclusion of comments upon the philosophical dimensions of foundational inquiry currently pursued in the science-based professions.

To begin with, philosophy is a humanistic discipline. Like languages and literature, but unlike the sciences, it focuses on what is distinctly human by definition: human thought and culture. It engages in reflection upon the assumed potential for and limitations of human knowledge and experience by offering forms of analysis and argumentation concerning foundational problems of knowledge, value, and being.

An especially interesting feature of the philosophical tradition is that it celebrates uniqueness. Philosophers place a high premium upon the uniqueness of the intellectual frameworks created to approach philosophical problems. They herald, also, novel forms of argumentation which frequently grow from these frameworks. Innovational frameworks and lines of argument are hallmarks of this tradition. This has led some philosophers to suggest that their role is to identify problems specifically outside of the discipline and to use philosophical approaches to analyze, argue, and offer solutions (Russell, 1950; Popper, 1962).

Other distinguishing features of this tradition are its reliance on argument and analysis. If philosophy could be said to have a method, a contention with which most philosophers would likely take umbrage, this method would best be portrayed as the development of various forms of intellectual analysis and argument. However, several

philosophers, after analysis and argument, have produced a philosophical vision which led them to designate a method of inquiry: notably, the
phenomenologist, Edmund Husserl (1970), and the pragmatist, John
Dewey (1938).

THE PHILOSOPHICAL TRADITION

From the time of the Ancient Greeks until the twentieth century,
philosophers, in the spirit of inquiry, raised questions concerning the
ultimate nature of the cosmos, society, and man. They reflected and
argued about the constituents and processes of reality, the meaning of
existence, the sources and validity of knowledge, the formal rules of
thought and inquiry, the standards of exemplary human conduct, the
criteria of beauty, and the ideal form of social organization. The formal
labels given these intellectual studies include *metaphysics*, *ontology*, *epistemology*, *logic*, *ethics*, *esthetics*, and *social philosophy*.

The most distinguished philosophers offered a series of consistent
answers to such clusters of questions, as mentioned above, creating a
reasoned synthesis or world view which, in the literature, have assumed
the status of "systems." Distinguished creators of philosophical systems,
at least in Western civilization, include Plato, Aristotle, Descartes,
Spinoza, Liebniz, Locke, Hume, Kant, and Hegel. Concurrently, many
of these philosophers also were major contributors to the development
of the discipline of mathematics (Kneak & Kneak, 1962; Temple, 1981).

By the twentieth century, however, the traditional approach of generating grand speculative systems drew severe criticism. The advent of the
natural and social sciences, with their distinctive empirical methodologies
for acquiring and evaluating knowledge claims, prompted many
philosophers to change their perspectives about the business of their
discipline (Bobik, 1970). Anglo-American philosophers, in particular,
saw the older tradition as far too speculative (Carnap, 1932; Ayer, 1936,
1959; Wittgenstein, 1961). Armchair reflection on the nature of reality
was thought dubious and misleading. Metaphysical speculation was attacked as creating illusions and proliferating strange entities. The development of verification procedures even led a prominent school of
philosophical thought, the Logical Positivists, to declare the only statements with meaning were those which were verifiable. Vigorous
philosophical discussions of the foundational problems of scientific
methodology ensued (Popper, 1935; Feigl & Brodbeck, 1953; Hanson,
1958; Natanson, 1963; Suppe, 1977; Phillips, 1987).

Advances in logic also encouraged shifts in philosophic outlook. In critical instances, Aristotelian logic was revealed to reflect, solely, a grammatical order that misrepresented true logical form: thereby necessitating the creation of a new, modern logic (Kneak & Kneak, 1962).

Charges that language itself carried deception stimulated interest in the analysis of language. The linguistic movement, which developed in this century, was dedicated to the discovery and solution of philosophic puzzles thought to be embedded in the uses of language. Some among the movement attempted to distance themselves from ordinary language, insisting on reconstruction through the creation of "ideal languages" (i.e., mathematical and logical symbolism, among other things) (Urmson, 1956; Rorty, 1967).

Meanwhile, in Europe, speculative philosophy was not altogether abandoned. What might be called "limited speculation" was championed in the works of the phenomenologists and the members of the Frankfurt School (Jay, 1973). These phenomenologists developed lines of speculative thought claimed to be presuppositionless. The Frankfurt School honored speculation as a characteristic of philosophic activity; however, they denied the speculative adequacy of previous traditional philosophic systems, as well as the suitability of the then current methodologies in the social sciences (Scruton, 1981). Hermeneutics, the discipline of contextual interpretation of documents extended in the twentieth century to the study of human action through specific context, also saw renewed interest (Gadamer, 1977; Phillips, 1987).

By the middle of this century, the discipline of philosophy reflected widespread disagreement as to the nature of philosophic inquiry.

METHODOLOGICAL APPROACHES

Methodologically speaking, philosophers primarily engage in argumentation. General patterns of argument which identify intellectual structures and organizations, state relationships, and convey consistent conclusions provide a modus operandi for philosophers. Although the body of their works frequently reflect diverse intellectual activities, such as the formulating of analysis, the drawing of distinctions, the discussion of assumptions, and the construction of interpretations, these specific activities may be construed, broadly, as forms of argument. That is, argumentation by analysis, argumentation by interpretation, and argumentation by logical stricture are specialized intellectual tools of the philosopher.

Argumentation by Analysis

In this century, argumentation by analysis has been associated with the language philosophers. Variously labeled "language analysis," "analytic philosophy," "philosophical analysis," and "conceptual analysis," users of this approach utilize no set pattern of analysis, but are in general agreement as to the focus of their enterprise; which is to disclose pseudo problems arising from the misuse of language (Urmson, 1956; Austin, 1961; Rorty, 1967). However, argumentation by analysis is hardly new. The older tradition, from which the language philosophers have tried to distance themselves, regularly engaged in analysis. This analysis frequently took the form of examining examples and making comparisons. By this view, Plato's myths may even be interpreted as "poetic analysis."

But what do these analyses have in common? Philosophical analyses are attempts to clarify thinking and meaning. The disclosure of ambiguity, the uncovering of assumptions, the discovery of inconsistencies, the identification of relevant distinctions make it possible, through analysis, to draw consistent conclusions about and between thought, language, and reality.

Argumentation by Interpretation

Another broad class of argument is argumentation by interpretation. Intellectual configurations of this form are harder to characterize. Sometimes these arguments are extensive and sweeping. In such cases, argumentation by interpretation is a measure of how an argument is rallied. The frameworks, organization, and sequencing form the internal structure. The strength of the intellectual message is based on the argument's development.

Often, argumentation by interpretation is a specialized intellectual vehicle aimed at giving breadth or background to an overall endeavor. In such cases, it may take the form of historical or sociological surveys (Swartz, Parkinson, & Edgerton, 1980). Literatures, past and present, may be reviewed and explored for positions taken by a series of authors or schools of individuals dedicated to particular theses. It is not uncommon to analyze the work of leading philosophers in a survey of this kind. Here, argumentation by interpretation is meant to bolster a thesis by providing assurance that a position has been maintained or held. In rather rare instances, the reviewer may trace the development of particular theses.

As every other philosophical system before it, argumentation by interpretation has had its critics (Feyerabend, 1963). Those philosophers enamored of a view of science which suggests that truth emerges only from close scrutiny of "facts," particularly, dislike interpretations. Misconstruing science as non-selective, non-interpretative, and conclusive, this group fails to see what the sciences and humanities have in common. And, again, interpretation, even now as a dilemma, rises here. Because science attempts to interpret the empirical, no pure facts exist. Theoretical constructions, which guide scientists to their interpretation of experience or reality, are intellectual instruments for interpretation before they are anything else. Moreover, scientists are as much caught up in problems surrounding language, categorical distinctions, and assumptions as scholars.

Argumentation by Logical Stricture

The final class of argument are those forms dominated by logical considerations. Simply put, logic is the application of principles to garner consistency in argument. Since arguments entail inference, logical rules are utilized to ensure validity in the process of reasoning. Discovering inconsistency, therefore, may be significant enough to consider as a major form of criticism. Fallacies, for instance, are incorrect forms of reasoning. Traditionally, logic focused its studies on what constituted proof or conclusive evidence. These logical studies were closely linked to the methodologies of the sciences (Cohen & Nagel, 1934). However, with the advent of concern over language and its misuse, arguments may center on any number of logical considerations within and outside the sciences.

PHILOSOPHIES OF SCIENCE

Studies in the philosophy of science and social science are a specialization in the discipline of philosophy. These studies take their beginnings, generally, from the work of Francis Bacon (1965). Bacon, who lived during the sixteenth century, was deeply concerned with the lack of an empirical method to ensure a proper investigation toward the revelation of truth. Reacting to the intellectual conditions of his cultural period, much of which he considered spurious, Bacon rejected forms of armchair speculation and reasoning. Loathing prejudices, abuses of language, and reliance on institutional sources for the authority of knowledge, Bacon raised the fundamental question of the scientific method itself by asking what it was. He answered this question by pointing out that science begins with observation and inducts to theoretical knowledge.

Interestingly, but consistently, Bacon focused on the researcher as the primary source of error. Bacon exhorted researchers to observe "purely," recording only what they found, and thus avoid contamination through preconceptions held by the researcher (Swartz, Perkinson, & Edgerton, 1980).

This Baconian empirical program, which continues to found interpretations of the "scientific method," remains a distinguished legacy. However, it is certainly *not* flawless. By the twentieth century, it became increasingly apparent that a researcher could not observe "purely" and must bring intellectual equipment to science in order to know, among other things, what to observe and how to observe it (Hanson, 1958; Popper, 1962; Scheffler, 1967; Wigner, 1967; Kuhn, 1970; Fodor, 1984). And, by mid-twentieth century, it became even clearer that the researcher must not only bring complex frameworks and methodological sophistication to science, but, also, considerable creativity.

Another area of disagreement with Bacon was his advocacy of inductive logic in the method of inquiry. Attacked first by David Hume (1888) in the eighteenth century, inductive logic has come under increased criticism, primarily by the philosopher of logic and scientific methodology, Karl R. Popper (1935, 1959, 1962). Popper has insisted, as Hume did, that inductive logic is rationally unjustifiable. Going further, however, he has argued that inductive logic underlies verification procedures, making this form of scientific testing extremely vulnerable to error.

Logical Positivism

Logical positivism is perhaps the most influential philosophy of science and social science in the twentieth century. Its major statement stems from the Vienna Circle, a group of philosophers and mathematicians under the influence of the philosopher Moritz Schlick. Many distinguished modern philosophers of science and social science have been associated with the development of this position (Bridgman, 1927; Carnap, 1932; Ayer, 1936; Hempel & Oppenheim, 1948; Feigl & Brodbeck, 1953; Bergman, 1958; Reichenbach, 1962). Its significance and influence may well be judged by the label its most recent and powerful critics gave it—"the Received View" (Suppe, 1977).

Logical Positivism is an attempt at rational reconstruction. By examining extant methods in physics and chemistry, these philosophers and mathematicians reconstructed the logical and empirical components of the structure of knowledge. Theories, explanations, concepts, and definitions were identified as parts of this structure. Rules were formulated for proper and adequate explanations (Popper, 1935; Hempel & Oppenheim, 1948; Pitt, 1988) and concept formation (Hempel, 1952), including, of course, operational definitions. Since the Logical Positivists argued that verifiability was the criterion of meaningfulness, these deductive structures were grounded in phenomenal conditions, or put simply, observational terms. Thus, Logical Positivists claimed that metaphysical entities, to them a major source of error in knowledge systems, would finally become unnecessary. Their elimination was hailed by Logical Positivists as an essential advance in human thought.

However, Logical Positivism has not escaped its critics and is currently under severe challenge. Led by the innovative work of Popper (1935, 1959, 1962, 1966, 1972, 1982, 1983), Kuhn (1970) and Feyerabend (1975, 1981) have offered alternative perspectives of the scientific enterprise. Raising the question, "How does our knowledge grow?" these philosophers of science have engaged in wide-ranging historical studies of the scientific milieu in which they work. Focusing on the actual practices of scientists, they have suggested numerous interpretations of scientific activity itself, and have opened the way for a previously unheralded questioning.

New Perspectives

Current understanding of scientific knowledge has developed from the work of the critics mentioned above. In their view, scientific knowledge grows through sophisticated forms of refinement which amount to "replacement" as opposed to a process of simple accumulation. That is, the vehicles leading to refinement of conceptual frameworks and theoretical networks, which also lead to accumulation through replacement, vary with particular views. Popper (1959) emphasizes formulating theory in an empirically testable structure, attempting to refute it, then utilizing negative outcomes to create revised conjectures. Since Popper sees knowledge as a human creation and researchers as creative but fallible, he directs scientists' attention to boldly conjecturing, then searching out error. Kuhn (1970) suggests scientists accumulate anomalies until skepticism of the scientific community gathers (at which time the anomalies are treated as refutations) leading to paradigm replacement. Paradigm shifts may take place, also, through advances in instrumentation. Feyerabend (1975, 1981) favors comparative testing among multiple frameworks, utilizing crucial tests and refutations to construct new frameworks. Details of these philosophies differ considerably; however, their arguments draw largely from historical precedents suggesting a re-interpretation of the history of science (Agassi, 1963; Kuhn, 1970). Opposition to these philosophical approaches may be found, among others, in the works of Lakatos (1970), Suppe (1977), and Shapere (1983).

The literature of the philosophy of science and social science may be viewed as a "meta" discussion of the assumptions of various approaches and methodologies of research. In professional literatures, such discussions are usually referred to in epistemological terms. These studies provide the humanistic cornerstone of scientific research programs. However, it is important to note that metaphysical issues are frequently intertwined with positions taken in the philosophy of science and social science. An example appropriate to the literature of nursing is found, for this author, in foundational discussions of holism.

FOUNDATIONAL RESEARCH AND RESEARCHER PREPARATION

Foundational research is methodical scholarly discussion of assumptions made in professional literatures. In the science-based professions, philosophers focus foundational research generally on conceptualizations which form the background knowledge to the scientific frameworks. This author has found that such background knowledge may or may not be articulated in the professional literature, however. Typically, philosophers call background knowledge into question when a clash emerges between the conceptual assumptions and components of the scientific framework (Popper, 1976). Philosophers may also prompt foundational discussions when the identifying conceptual foundations which conflict with one another suddenly appear crucial to changes in the scientific framework. Occasionally, scientific researchers formulate new problems that call for new methodologies and thereby prompt foundational discussion. Whether foundational inquiries are prompted by philosopher or scientific researcher, they are used to articulate, clarify, and refine basic conceptualizations. Traditionally, philosophical analysis has served as the method for such investigations and debates that lead to reconceptualization, and, ultimately, intellectual consistency between background knowledge and scientific frameworks (Breines, 1986; Sarter, 1988).

To engage in foundational research requires appropriate educational preparation, which may vary according to the dimensions of the foundational problem being addressed. Essential to foundational research is a strong intellectual grasp of the professional literature as well as a complete understanding of the professional literature in the specific problem area associated with the foundational inquiry. The needed comprehension may include historical literacy surrounding the problem of investigation. Since forms of uniqueness play a prominent role in foundational studies of a philosophical nature, learning to fashion an argument based on exploratory studies and analysis is a requisite skill. Specific preparation may involve philosophical course work and extensive reading. A general background in philosophical discussions is helpful in acquiring the skills relevant to comprehending methodological moves and the rules associated with them. Fledglings, perhaps, learn this most readily by a study of exemplary predecessors, more specifically, by a study of the methodological moves of the argument or analysis at hand rather than the particular intellectual content.

It is frequently said by professional philosophers that the outcome of a philosophical education is not so much learning philosophy but learning to philosophize. This is as true of foundational studies of a philosophical nature as it is of philosophy proper.

REFERENCES

Agassi, J. (1963). *Towards an historiography of science.* The Hague, Netherlands: Mouton.

Austin, J. (1961). *Philosophical papers.* Oxford: The Clarendon Press.

Ayer, A. (1936). *Language, truth and logic.* (2nd ed.). London: Gollanez.

Ayer, A. (Ed.). (1959). *Logical positivism.* Glencoe, IL: Free Press.

Bergman, G. (1958). *Philosophy of science.* Madison, WI: University of Wisconsin Press.

Bobik, J. (Ed.). (1970). *The nature of philosophical inquiry.* Notre Dame: The University of Notre Dame Press.

Breines, E. (1986). *Origins and adaptations: A philosophy of practice.* Lebanon, NJ: Geri-Rehab., Inc.

Bridgeman, P. W. (1927). *The logic of modern physics.* New York: Macmillan Press.

Carnap, R. (1959). The elimination of metaphysics through the logical analysis of language. In A. J. Ayer (Ed.), *Logical positivism.* Glencoe, IL: Free Press.

Cohen, M., & Nagel, E. (1934). *An introduction to logic and scientific method.* New York: Harcourt, Brace and Company.

Dewey, J. (1938). *Logic: The study of inquiry.* New York: Henry Holt & Co.

Feigl, H., & Brodbeck, M. (Eds.). (1953). *Readings in the philosophy of science.* New York: Appleton-Century-Crofts.

Feyerabend, P. (1963). How to be a good empiricist: A plea for tolerance in matters epistemological. In P. H. Nidditch (Ed.), *The philosophy of science* (pp. 12–39). Oxford: Oxford University Press.

Feyerabend, P. (1975). *Against method: Outline of an anarchistic theory of knowledge.* London: New Left Books.

Feyerabend, P. (1981). *Realism, rationalism, and scientific method. Philosophical Papers, Vol. I.* New York: Cambridge University Press.

Feyerabend, P. (1981). *Problems of empiricism. Philosophical Papers, Vol. II.* New York: Cambridge University Press.

Fodor, J. (1984). Observation reconsidered. *Philosophy of Science, 51,* 23–43.

Gadamer, H. (1977). *Philosophical hermeneutics.* (E. Linge, Trans.). Berkeley: University of California Press.

Hanson, N. R. (1958). *Patterns of discovery.* Cambridge: Cambridge University Press.

Hempel, C., & Oppenheim, P. (1948). The logic of explanation. In H. Feigl & M. Brodbeck (Eds.), *Readings in the philosophy of science* (pp. 319–352). New York: Appleton-Century-Crofts.

Hempel, C. G. (1952). Fundamentals of concept formation. In *International encyclopedia of unified science.* Chicago: University of Chicago Press.

Husserl, E. (1970). *Logical investigations.* (J. N. Findlay, Trans.). London: Routledge, and Kegan Paul.

Jay, M. (1973). *The dialectical imagination: A history of the Frankfurt school and the institute of social research, 1923-1950.* Boston: Little Brown & Co.

Kneak, W., & Kneak, M. (1962). *The development of logic.* Oxford: The Clarendon Press.

Kuhn, T. (1970). The structure of scientific revolutions. (2nd. ed.) In *International encyclopedia of unified science.* Chicago: University of Chicago Press.

Lakatos, I. (1970). Falsification and the methodology of scientific research programs. In I. Lakatos & A. Musgrave (Eds.), *Criticism and the growth of scientific knowledge* (pp. 91–196). London: Cambridge University Press.

Natanson, M. (Ed.). (1963). *Philosophy of science.* New York: Random House.

Phillips, D. C. (1987). *Philosophy, science and social inquiry: Contemporary methodological controversies in social science and related applied fields of research.* New York: Pergamon Press.

Pitt, J. (Ed.). (1988). *Theories of explanation.* New York: Oxford University Press.

Popper, K. (1935). *Logik der forschung.* Wien: J. Springer.

Popper, K. (1959). *The logic of scientific discovery.* London: Hutchinson.

Popper, K. (1962). *Conjectures and refutations.* London: Routledge and Kegan Paul.

Popper, K. (1966). *The open society and its enemies* (5th ed. rev.). London: Routledge and Kegan Paul.

Popper, K. (1972). *Objective knowledge.* Oxford: Clarendon Press.

Popper, K. (1976). The myth of the framework. In E. Frieman (Ed.), *The abdication of philosophy: Philosophy and the public good.* LaSalle, IL: Open Court.

Popper, K. (1982). *Quantum theory and the schism in physics: From the postscript to the logic of scientific discovery.* Totowa: Rowman & Littlefield.

Popper, K. (1983). *Realism and the aim of science: From the postscript to the logic of scientific discovery.* Totowa: Rowman and Littlefield.

Popper, K. (1983). *The open universe: An argument for indeterminism: From the postscript to the logic of scientific discovery.* Totowa: Rowman & Littlefield.

Reichenbach, H. (1962). *The rise of scientific philosophy.* Berkeley: University of California Press.

Rorty, R. (Ed.). (1967). *The linguistic turn.* Chicago: University of Chicago Press.

Russell, B. (1950). *Unpopular essays.* New York: Simon and Schuster.

Sarter, B. (1988). *The stream of becoming: A study of Martha Roger's theory.* New York: The National League for Nursing.

Scheffler, I. (1967). *Science and subjectivity.* Indianapolis, IN: Bobbs-Merrill.

Scruton, R. (1981). *From Descartes to Wittgenstein: A short history of modern philosophy.* New York: Harper & Row.

Shapere, D. (1983). *Reason and the search for knowledge.* Dordecht, Holland: Reidel.

Suppe, F. (1977). *The structure of scientific theories* (2nd ed.). Urbana, IL: University of Illinois Press.

Swartz, R., Perkinson, H., & Edgerton, S. (1980). *Knowledge and fallibilism: Essays on improving education.* New York: New York University Press.

Temple, G. (1981). *100 Years of mathematics.* London: Duckworth Press.

Urmson, J. (1956). *Philosophical analysis: Its development between the two wars.* Oxford: Clarendon Press.

Wigner, E. P. (1967). *Symmetries and reflections.* Bloomington, IN: Indiana University Press.

Wittgenstein, L. (1961). *Tractatus logico-philosophicus.* (D. F. Pears & B. F. McGuinness, Trans.). London: Routledge and Kegan Paul.

BIBLIOGRAPHY

Achinstein, P. (1968). *Concepts of science.* Baltimore: Johns Hopkins Press.

Achinstein, P., & Barker, S. (1969). *The legacy of logical positivism.* Baltimore: Johns Hopkins Press.

Agassi, J. (1968). *The continuing revolution: A history of physics from the Greeks to Einstein.* New York: McGraw-Hill Book Company.

Agassi, J. (1977). *Towards a rational philosophical anthropology.* The Hague, Netherlands: Martinus Nijhoff.

Bacon, F. (1965). *Selected writings.* New York: Schocken Books.

Bacon, F. (1978). *Novum organum.* Oxford: Clarendon Press.

Blanchard, B. (1954). *On philosophical style.* Bloomington, IN: Indiana University Press.

Bohm, D. (1976). *Fragmentation and wholeness.* Jerusalem: Van Leer Foundation.

Bohm, D. (1980). *Wholeness and the implicate order*. London: Routledge and Kegan Paul.

Bridgman, P. W. (1927). *The logic of modern physics*. New York: Macmillan.

Brodbeck, M. (Ed.). (1968). *Readings in the philosophy of the social sciences*. New York: Macmillan.

Campbell, D. (1978). Qualitative knowing and action research. In M. Brenner & P. March (Eds.), *The social context of method*. New York: St. Martin's Press.

Carnap, R. (1967). *The logical structure of the world: Pseudo problems in philosophy* (R. A. George, Trans.). Berkeley: University of California Press.

Edgerton, S. (1967, May). Learning by induction. *Social education*, 1–13.

Edgerton, S. (1969). Is there a scientific method? *History of Education Quarterly, IX*, 492–496.

Edgerton, S. (1973). The technological imagination: A philosopher looks at nursing. *Journal of thought, 8*, 57–65.

Edgerton, S. (1981). What is a model? Modeling and the professions. In S. Wagner and W. Geeslin (Eds.), *Modeling mathematical cognitive development* (pp. 1–10). Columbus, OH: ERIC Clearinghouse for Science, Mathematics and Environmental Education.

Gadamer, H. (1981). *Reason in the age of science*. Cambridge, MA: MIT Press.

Gellner, E. (1963). *Words and things: A critical account of linguistic philosophy and a study of ideology*. London: Gollancz.

Gellner, E. (1964). *Thought and change*. London: Weidenfeld & Nicolson.

Glaser, B., & Strauss, A. (1967). *The discovery of grounded theory: Strategies for qualitative research*. Chicago: Aldine.

Gutting, G. (Ed.). (1980). *Paradigms and revolutions: Applications and appraisals of Thomas Kuhn's philosophy of science*. Notre Dame: University of Notre Dame Press.

Habermas, J. (1972). *Knowledge and human interests*. (J. Shapiro, Trans.). London: Heinemann.

Habermas, J. (1973). *Theory and practice*. (J. Viertel, Trans.). Boston: Beacon Press.

Hacking, I. (Ed.). (1981). *Scientific revolutions*. New York: Oxford University Press.

Hayek, F. (1955). *The counter-revolution of science: Studies on the abuses of reason*. London: The Free Press of Glencoe.

Hume, D. (1888). A treatise of human nature. Oxford: Clarendon Press.

Kent, R. (1981). *The politics of social theory: Habermas, Freud, and the critique of positivism*. Chicago: The University of Chicago Press.

Larson, M. S. (1977). *The rise of professionalism: A sociological analysis*. Berkeley: The University of California Press.

Laudan, L. (1978). *Progress and its problems: Toward a theory of scientific growth*. Berkeley: University of California Press.

Levinson, P. (Ed.). (1982). *In pursuit of truth: Essays in honor of Karl Popper's 80th birthday*. New Jersey: The Humanities Press.

McCarthy, T. (1978). *The critical theory of Jurgen Habermas.* Cambridge: MIT Press.

Medawar, P. (1979). *Advice to a young scientist.* New York: Harper & Row.

Medawar, P. (1982). *Pluto's republic.* Oxford: Oxford University Press.

Medawar, P. (1984). *The limits of science.* New York: Harper & Row.

Nidditch, P. H. (Ed.). (1968). *The philosophy of science.* Oxford: Oxford University Press.

Nishiyama, C., & Leube, K. (Eds.). (1984). *The essence of Hayek.* Stanford, CA: Hoover Institution Press.

Passmore, J. (1961). *Philosophical reasoning.* London: Gerald Duckworth and Co., Ltd.

Phillips, D. C. (1976). *Holistic thought in social science.* Stanford, CA: Stanford University Press.

Polanyi, M. (1958). *Personal knowledge.* Chicago: University of Chicago Press.

Popper, K., & Eccles, J. (1977). *The self and its brain: An argument for interactionism.* New York: Springer-Verlag.

Robinson, D. N. (1979). *Systems of modern psychology: A critical sketch.* New York: Columbia University Press.

Rose, G. (1978). *The melancholy science: An introduction to the thought of Theodore W. Adorno.* New York: Columbia University Press.

Rosenberg, C. E. (1978). *No other gods: On science and American social thought.* Baltimore: Johns Hopkins University Press.

Rothstein, W. (1972). *American physicians in the nineteenth century: From sects to science.* Baltimore: Johns Hopkins University Press.

Russell, B., & Whitehead, A. (1910). *Principia mathematica.* Cambridge: Cambridge University Press.

Schillp, P. (Ed.). (1974). *The philosophy of Karl Popper.* LaSalle, IL: Open Court.

Schon, D. (1983). *The reflective practitioner: How professionals think in action.* New York: Basic Books, Inc.

Sloan, D. (Ed.). (1981). *Toward the recovery of wholeness: Knowledge, education, and human values.* New York: Teachers College Press.

Smith, J. (1983). *The idea of health: Implications for the nursing professional.* New York: Teachers College Press.

Spiegelberg, H. (1965). *The phenomenological movement.* (2 vols.). The Hague, Netherlands: Martinus Nijhoff.

Suppe, F., & Jacox, A. K. (1985). Philosophy of science and the development of nursing theory. In H. H. Wesley and J. J. Fitzpatrick (Eds.), *Annual review of nursing research* (Vol. 3), (pp. 241–267). New York: Springer Publishing Company.

Urbach, P. (1987). *Francis Bacon's philosophy of science: An account and a reappraisal.* LaSalle, IL: Open Court.

Wartofsky, M. (1968). *Conceptual foundations of scientific thought: An introduction to the philosophy of science.* New York: Macmillan.

Winch, P. (1967). *The idea of a social science.* London: Routledge and Kegan Paul.

Windelband, W. (1893). *A history of philosophy: The formation and development of its problems and conceptions.* (J. Tufts, Trans.). New York: Macmillan.

Wittgenstein, L. (1958). *Philosophical investigations* (3rd ed.), (G. E. M. Anscombe, Trans.). New York: Macmillan.

Metaphysical Analysis

Barbara Sarter

In its broadest sense, philosophy is the process and expression of rational reflection upon experience (Hastings, 1961). Bertrand Russell (1945) describes philosophy as something intermediate between theology and science: "All *definite* knowledge—so I should contend—belongs to science; all *dogma* as to what surpasses definite knowledge belongs to theology" (p. xiii). Why then study problems for which there are no definite solutions? There are many compelling reasons for doing so. Since the beginning of human self-awareness and conscious reflection, persons have developed theories of the world and human life which have profoundly influenced the way they conducted their lives. Whether one is aware of it or not, every person, in a sense, is a philosopher, and every field of human activity, including nursing, is based on an implicit set of philosophical assumptions about the nature of its domain.

Further, although definite or complete answers may not be possible through philosophical thinking alone, our answers may become more complete and accurate through the application of reason or intuition to experience. As our experience of the universe expands through scientific and personal avenues, it is imperative that our philosophical thinking likewise expand. Science and philosophy must develop in harmony, for together they can provide us with a more complete understanding of the world than either one alone. But are science and philosophy compatible?

Hutchison (1977) distinguishes science from philosophy in terms of their range of context. Whereas science deals with a limited and specific reality (the material world), philosophy, traditionally, and metaphysics, in particular, encompasses "all-inclusive totality"—the entire universe, which includes the material world as a matter of course. Additionally, the classical goals of philosophical thinking are *clarification* of philosophic issues embedded in our common humanity; *perspective* so that one sees oneself as part of the larger universe; and articulation and appraisal of *values* that define and sustain our humanity.

As one of the traditional branches of philosophy, the task of metaphysics is to explore the most fundamental problems of knowledge and reality. Its primary activity is the investigation of the essential nature of reality as a whole. Throughout the ages a number of recurrent metaphysical issues have emerged, including: unity versus multiplicity, being versus becoming, potentiality versus actuality, order versus disorder, the universal versus the particular, appearance versus reality, matter versus spirit, the nature of causality, and the existence of values in the universe as a whole. Reflection upon these issues reveals that metaphysics is perhaps the most fundamental of the branches of philosophy, for one's position on these issues will guide one's thinking in all other philosophical domains, such as logic, ethics, epistemology, and esthetics.

Of equal significance is the fundamental importance of these issues to scientific endeavor, including nursing science. Nursing defines its domain and its practice on the basis of a number of metaphysical assumptions, whether we leave them implicit or make them explicit. A careful analysis of the variety of nursing theories (Sarter, 1988), research methods, and approaches to practice shows that the same assumptions are not held by all the members of the discipline. This provides an important justification for nursing scholars to engage in metaphysical analysis. Donaldson and Crowley (1978) presented a clear and widely embraced mandate to the profession when they maintained that "a discipline is characterized by a unique perspective, a distinct way of viewing all phenomena, which ultimately defines the limits and nature of its inquiry" (p. 113). This unique disciplinary perspective, commonly called a metaparadigm, is yet to be fully attained in nursing, and metaphysics has an important role to play in its achievement.

HISTORICAL OVERVIEW OF METAPHYSICS

Humility is an appropriate sentiment for the novice approaching metaphysics. It is prudent to begin by studying the great world philosophers and systems. Such a study will provide a necessary foundation for the application of metaphysical analysis to a practice discipline.

Western philosophers identify the classical Greek era as marking the beginning of metaphysical speculation. This belief betrays ignorance of the highly sophisticated and complex philosophical systems of ancient India, which undoubtedly influenced the early Greek philosophers. Vedic philosophy found its most subtle and refined expression in the Upanishads, which were recorded by rishis or "seers" who left no personal signatures. To this day, the Upanishads are held in utmost respect and are felt to express the earliest and most profound philosophical insights into the nature of reality. The exact dates are not known, but it is agreed that their recording occurred prior to the sixth century B.C. (Hiriyanna, 1932). The Upanishads, totalling 12 major and over 200 minor works, describe the ultimate reality as unitary and spiritual in nature.

Six major systems of Indian philosophy emerged after the appearance of the Upanishads, expressing virtually the full range of metaphysical speculation later encountered in Western philosophy: from materialism to spiritualism, dualism to monism, becoming to being. Buddhism, for example, began as a religion and later became a philosophy as a defense against Hinduism and Jainism (Hiriyanna, 1932).

Aristotle (1952) was the first to use the term metaphysics in a purely descriptive manner since the treatise so named was placed above or before his treatise on physics. He described his endeavor as follows: "The most intelligible matters are first principles and basic reasons, since it is by and through them that any given subject becomes intelligible, not vice versa . . . the knowledge we are seeking . . . is the theory of first principles and reasons" (pp. 7–8). Aristotle called this knowledge "wisdom," and maintained that wisdom consists of such theoretical rather than practical knowledge. His statement of the problems to be explored in metaphysics set the format of metaphysical discussion for centuries to follow.

It was not until the modern scientific revolution that Aristotle's world view was largely set aside. Aristotle explored the issues of unity versus multiplicity, being versus becoming, universals versus particulars, appearance versus reality, and the nature of causality. His theory of causality is of particular relevance to the human sciences, though it has suffered complete rejection by the physical sciences. Briefly, Aristotle described four kinds of causality: material, relating to the substance of an entity; efficient, relating to immediately preceding events; formal, relating to the "form" or essence of an entity; and final, relating to the goal or final result of an entity or process. Inherent in the last two kinds of causality is the teleological view that an organism's potentiality exerts a causal influence on the course of its development.

Plato, another important influence in metaphysical thought throughout the Middle Ages, maintained that a realm entirely separate from the material world exists, the realm of true Reality and eternal Ideas or

Forms of which the world of human experience is merely a shadow. Greek philosophers even earlier than Plato had engaged in metaphysical speculation, some of which is remarkably relevant to modern scientific understanding. For example, Democritus and other atomists believed that the universe consists of minute invisible units of matter in a state of constant motion.

Spinoza, Leibniz, and Hegel, ranging from the eighteenth to the nineteenth centuries, were later giants of Western metaphysics. They developed complex metaphysical systems depicting a relatively static and highly organized universe.

However, with the dawn of the scientific revolution and its concern with observation as the source of knowledge, these grand metaphysical systems assumed a secondary place in philosophy. And, as logical positivism and its method of linguistic analysis assumed precedence in academic philosophy, metaphysics was rejected entirely as a meaningless philosophical activity because it failed the test of verifiability (Ayer, 1946). Contemporary philosophers of the analytic tradition admit, however, that even positivism rests upon a set of metaphysical assumptions about the nature of reality, thus making metaphysics seemingly an inescapable foundation of all intellectual activity (Hutchison, 1977).

The Darwinian view of evolution as a temporal process stimulated a new force in metaphysics—that of "process philosophy." Twentieth-century philosophers such as Whitehead and Teilhard de Chardin developed views of the universe as continuously evolving toward higher levels of consciousness, a perspective which was first stated millenia earlier by the Vedic *rishis*. These philosophers have exerted a significant influence on theories of nursing currently under development and testing (Sarter, 1988). This brings us directly to the issue of the relevance of metaphysics to the discipline of nursing.

METAPHYSICS AND NURSING

Relevance to Nursing

A number of specific metaphysical issues are directly relevant to nursing theory and nursing science. One issue most urgently in need of exploration is that of reductionism versus holism. Nursing theorists have assumed differing positions on this issue, ranging from Rogers' insistence that the whole *cannot* be understood through examination of its parts to Johnson's breakdown of human beings into systems. Analysis of this issue requires exploration of biophilosophy, the discipline which addresses philosophical problems related to living organisms.

Another critical area for metaphysical analysis in nursing is the nature of human life and personhood. What is the ontological status of human life—its meaning and purpose, if any, in the universe? What is the status of free will and human agency? What, if any, is the reason for human suffering and the meaning of death? These questions have more than academic significance to nurses whose practice brings them into daily encounters with the heights and depths of human experience. Related to questions concerning the nature of human life is, of course, the nature of the universe as a whole—cosmology. Is there any fundamental order or purpose in the universe, or are there only random events underlying the seeming order? Rogerian theory describes the universe as evolutionary, in a process of continuous change toward increasing diversity and negentropy, and also maintains that reality is four-dimensional. These are profound and, to some, radical, metaphysical statements based on, but not limited to, scientific knowledge. Other nursing theorists base their views on less explicit metaphysical assumptions which are equally in need of clarification and critique.

The body/mind or matter/spirit issue encompasses a number of exceedingly important questions for nursing theory, research, and practice. Are there any such separate entities or forces, or are they simply manifestations of one underlying reality? Or, is only matter real or only mind/spirit real? The implications of these questions for nursing, again, are profound. It appears that current thinking in health care is shifting away from a purely material view of human life and health toward views that acknowledge the reality of mind and spirit. These are complex philosophical areas which require rigorous analysis by nursing scholars so that their relevance to the discipline can be explored.

Still another set of metaphysical issues which have been addressed by recent nursing theorists, albeit in a philosophically unsophisticated manner, is that dealing with space, time, and causality (Sarter, 1988). Traditional empirical research is based on certain assumptions about space, time, and causality. Currently, both philosophers of science and metaphysicians are questioning these assumptions. The dramatic increase in the use of qualitative research methods in nursing demonstrates that the old assumptions are under attack here as well; yet the task of developing more appropriate metaphysical foundations for nursing science is still in its infancy. It should also be clear after this review of issues relevant to nursing that metaphysics has a critical role to play in all aspects of the discipline of nursing—theory, research, practice, and education.

Researcher Preparation

The nursing scholar who is interested in conducting metaphysical analysis—by either developing a new metaphysical foundation for nursing theory or in analyzing those which have been implied by other theorists—must first become familiar with the metaphysical thought of past and current philosophers. Coursework in philosophy and a willing mentor are extremely helpful. Through the study of the thought of others, the major metaphysical issues and problems, and the ways philosophers have dealt with them throughout the ages, will become evident. Some of the great histories of Western philosophy which are particularly valuable in gaining this perspective include those by Fuller (1955), Hoffding (1955), and Russell (1945). Of these, Russell's is indispensible. Primary works by the great metaphysicians must be read as well. For an essential review of Eastern metaphysics, the works by Hiriyanna (1932) and Sharma (1976) are invaluable. A number of significant works exploring the metaphysical implications of modern scientific knowledge exist and provide highly relevant perspectives. Harris (1983) provides a particularly thought-provoking study. Taylor's (1974) introduction to metaphysics has become a useful book for those who are unfamiliar with this branch of philosophy.

A close and repeated reading and analysis of the works of current nursing theorists is also an essential task. It is particularly revealing to study nursing theories in the light of one's newly acquired philosophical background. Problems, relevant issues, and philosophical flaws of nursing theory emerge. The researcher can then select a particular metaphysical problem or theme to focus on, or may feel that an entirely new approach to the metaphysical foundation of nursing theory is the goal.

Conducting the Research

As with any research method, the first—and, for many, the most difficult—step is to identify a researchable problem. As just indicated, the historical review and analysis of current nursing theory will suggest numerous problems worthy of investigation. Determining the scope of the research study is an important decision which will affect what problem is selected. In general, a specific problem or issue such as those mentioned earlier should be identified for analysis, rather than an all-encompassing question. The amount of time available for the project is a critical factor here, as well as the sophistication of the researcher.

Two areas traditionally explored by metaphysical analysis are ontology and teleology. Ontology deals with the nature of the real in its essence;

that is, in abstraction from its specific manifestations. The philosophical issues identified earlier in this chapter are largely ontological in character. From these one may select a particular question for analysis. The nature of the physical world, the nature of man, the relationship between the two, the ontological status of non-physical events, and the nature and status of consciousness are examples of appropriate ontological problems for nursing scholars to explore. Teleological problems deal with the question of purpose, goals, values, and meaning in the universe. What is the purpose or meaning of human life? How do health and illness relate to this meaning? Is the evolutionary process value-laden or goal-oriented? Is human development likewise purposeful? These are some relevant teleological issues for nursing.

The question selected for study will determine the particular approach to be taken in answering it. In most cases, a metaphysical study will require a review of past and current philosophical thought on the issue. This may be a global review or may involve the selection of representative works which reflect opposing points of view. Argument through interpretation is one primary mode of discussion in philosophical research (Edgerton, 1980). It is important to present all major positions taken on the question, to interpret and critically analyze these varying points of view, and then to justify the position taken by the researcher according to a specific set of criteria.

The criteria used to justify the conclusions drawn by the researcher may vary. The validity of the proposed view may be derived from its explanatory power. Does it explain most of the world as it is known and experienced by human beings? The comprehensiveness of the answer may also be cited in its defense. Coherence is another important criterion of the "truth" of a philosophical position. Do all the parts of the system of ideas set forth fit together logically? Do the individual elements reflect the overall meaning of the system? Esthetic criteria such as elegance and simplicity may also be used. Pragmatic criteria, whether the proposed position will prove to be useful in the sphere of practice, often are used to justify a point of view, as well. In addition to internal consistency, external consistency is essential. It is rarely justifiable to support a philosophical position which radically conflicts with universally accepted scientific facts. Of course, divergence may come in the *interpretation* of those facts, which may then reflect back upon the nature of those "facts" and their supposed immutability.

Edgerton (1980) identifies a number of essential elements for the evaluation of philosophical research. Because they are relevant to metaphysical analysis, they are listed below:

1. Is the topic to be explored explicitly identified early in the study?
2. Are the purposes and aims of the inquiry, as well as the methodology to be used, clearly stated early in the study?
3. Is the rationale for the study convincing? Is the study useful and generative of new insights?
4. Is the organization of the inquiry logical?
5. Is the major mode of discussion argumentation through interpretation rather than through empirical evidence?
6. Are the researcher's biases and personal perspective acknowledged if they are likely to influence interpretation of the literature and supporting evidence?
7. Are all major writings in the question or topic, both pro and con, consulted in the presentation of possible points of view? If not, is the rationale for selection of specific authors provided?
8. Is there consistency in the use of rhetoric and preservation of the selected authors' views in context throughout the study?
9. Are the strengths and weaknesses of opposing positions explicitly discussed in the argumentation of the researcher?
10. Are the underlying assumptions and presuppositions of the major positions explored identified?
11. Do the arguments developed in the inquiry adhere to the assumptions of the positions from which they were derived?
12. Are the intended readers of the study identified?
13. Is the proposed answer to the question intelligible and convincing to the intended readers?
14. Are the aims and purposes of the study accomplished?

CONCLUSION

Metaphysical analysis is a task which has largely been left to professional philosophers. Such professionals may question the validity of designating this as an appropriate research method for other academic disciplines. When this method is utilized by nursing scholars, it becomes a case of applied philosophy, and in this sense it is highly appropriate for scholars within the discipine of nursing to explore answers to significant philosophical questions which affect their knowledge domain.

As nursing begins to establish its significance as a human science, it becomes imperative that its philosophical foundation be developed. Metaphysics, if accepted as the science of "first principles," should form the foundation of nursing's metaparadigm. With a commonly shared metaphysical stance, the development of nursing theory, of appropriate research methods, and of a clear professional ethic may proceed without major internal conflict. Many current nursing theories have suggested, either implicitly or explicitly, particular, and often conflicting, metaphysical positions (Sarter, 1988). However, these positions are not always carefully developed in the manner described above. One major task of nursing scholarship is to insist that our theories flow from a sophisticated and clearly articulated philosophical foundation. The method of metaphysical analysis is indispensable for accomplishing this goal.

REFERENCES

Artistotle. (1952). *Metaphysics* (R. Hope, Trans.). Ann Arbor: University of Michigan.

Ayer, A. J. (1946). *Language, truth and logic.* New York: Dover.

Donaldson, S. K., & Crowley, D. M. (1978). The discipline of nursing. *Nursing Outlook 27*, 346–351.

Edgerton, S. (1980). Philosophical inquiry. Class notes, New York University, unpublished.

Fuller, B. A. G. (1955). *A history of philosophy* (3rd ed.). New York: Henry Holt.

Harris, E. (1983). *The foundations of metaphysics in science.* Lanham, MD: University Press of America.

Hastings, J. (Ed.). (1961). *Encyclopedia of religion and ethics.* New York: Scribner.

Hiriyanna, M. (1932). *Outlines of Indian philosophy.* London: George Allen & Unwin.

Hoffding, H. (1955). *A history of modern philosophy* (B. E. Meyer, Trans.). New York: Dover.

Hutchison, J. (1977). *Living options in world philosophy.* Honolulu: University Press of Hawaii.

Russell, B. (1945). *A history of western philosophy.* New York: Simon & Schuster.

Sarter, B. (1988). Philosophical sources of nursing theory. *Nursing Science Quarterly 1*(2).

Sharma, C. (1976). *A critical survey of Indian philosophy.* New Delhi: Motilal Banarsidass.

Taylor, R. (1974). *Metaphysics.* Englewood Cliffs, NJ: Prentice-Hall.

Hermeneutics

Francelyn Reeder

Hermeneutics comes from the Greek word, "hermeneia," which according to Klemm (1983), proposes three directions of meaning: "to express/expression, to interpret/interpretation (in the sense of clarify by commentary), and to translate/translation" (p. 18). In its earliest conception, hermeneutics was a department of exegetical theology (science and theory of literary interpretation). As such, hermeneutics established the principles which exegesis applies.

The more recent interest in hermeneutical dimensions of science concerns understanding and interpretation as processes (epistemology) and modes of being (ontology). The focus is not only on literary texts but has come to include history, art, symbol and myth, and human action.

Hermeneutics, therefore, has emerged as a promising resource for the social sciences. Recently, nursing scholars have argued convincingly for integration of quantitative and qualitative research methods from the standpoint of hermeneutics (Schultz, 1987a,b; Benoliel, 1987; Allen, 1985) and studies have implemented such a blending with seeming success (Allen, 1985; Davidson, 1988).

Explorations into the origin, history, and philosophical roots of hermeneutics provide the conceptual and pragmatic reasons why this ancient discipline, ever renewed, is relevant for nursing science and art today. It should not be surprising to discover in the humanities that curious minds across time have shared the impelling motive for understanding the present through recovery of the past (language and culture); but, for this author, a personal "re-cognition" was also a delightful surprise.

In addition, an in-depth return to the familiar skills of reading, writing, and speaking has revealed a profound human nexus in which understanding is made possible. The philosophical anthropologist, Max Scheler (1962), once said that language itself is the most integral characteristic of human beings and requires the involvement of both body and mind to accomplish its expression. Quantitative and qualitative distinctions in research "pale" in the face of this reminder and encourage their integration with due respect for the nature of language as human expression. Thus, a basic assumption underlying hermeneutics is that language possesses its own reality and power while referencing the world in which we live.

This rich insight, that language is not simply a tool that we manipulate but rather a medium on which we stand and out of which we are created, provides an awesome focus for any science or art. From this focus, and within the traditions of hermeneutics, ontological positions and epistemological approaches have developed with a central theme common to each: that understanding itself is an art and a science; a product and a process; a standpoint and a viewpoint. Because of the universality and versatility within the hermeneutic tradition, its applicability can be seen in philosophy, ethics, social sciences, history, the arts, rhetoric, literary writing and poetry, anthropology, biblical exegesis and, most recently, critical social theory. Nurse scholars have extended hermeneutical understanding to meaningful action in the context of practice (Benner, 1984; Berrey, 1987; Thompson, 1987; Allen, 1985; Allen, Benner, & Diekelmann, 1986), as well as theory development (Davidson, 1988; Smerke, 1988).

This chapter, then, provides an overview and illustration of central themes and strategies common to hermeneutics with the understanding that conceptual and pragmatic choices for nursing research will be enhanced through the power of language.

DEFINITION AND DESCRIPTION OF HERMENEUTICS

What is hermeneutics? The following analogy applies: Hermeneutics is like a road map for understanding the terrain of language; the signs of spoken and written expressions point out connections between the speaker or writer and the world in which he or she lives. On a map, you read "you are here" marked with a colored flag. The sign is meant to provide a reference point to locate yourself in relation to the region. This existential position enables you to make plans and think about further possibilities for your trip. Then you make choices and actualize some of the options available.

The person who constructed the map has experienced the region and obtained a sense of what might be helpful to strangers in finding their way. Each person, in fact, could use the map on different days with different goals and travel to different sites on the terrain as they prefer. If the location and map are in simple correspondence to each other and the signs used have one literal meaning, then anyone, even a child, can read it without great difficulty. Universal road signs and those in airports and restaurants are other examples of literal signs. Hermeneutic rules are not necessary for their interpretation. Basic reading skills of a common language and culture are sufficient.

However, if the map is of mountain terrain and is designed for mountain climbers, the signs will not have immediate reference to one peak or valley, nor to one trail or ravine, but rather to less obvious classifications appropriate for this type of terrain.

For example, one sign may refer to altitude, one to riverbeds, another to timberline, one to lake regions, and one to glaciers. Therefore, each sign has to be interpreted by the mountain climber with a typology and taxonomy directly related to the nature of mountains; it has to include signs for all of the possible attributes of mountains if the climber is to comprehend the area adequately to enable the most effective and enjoyable navigation of the mountain.

Accordingly, the signs will require that the climber possess more sophisticated reading skills (linguistic skills of interpretation) and a common language of mountaineering. This level of interpretation uses signs that have general double meanings. Reading for literal meaning would be inadequate here. Adequate interpretation will depend upon the events and meaning the climber gives to them as well as the sense and reference of the language used to express that experience.

In actuality, then, when the climber embarks on "this trail," he or she is experiencing an *event*; when he or she says, "this is Trail Ridge Mountain," he or she has made an existential reference at this time and place in his or her life. Further, when he or she says, "this is my favorite trail," the sense of this trail is expressed in a personal context; but because the climber has expressed this sense for others to hear, the exclamation has public meaning for anyone who can hear or read and who possesses the common language of the speaker to understand it.

Understanding itself is a common experience to us all. Yet it still remains formidable for just as many of us. Communication involves sending and receiving messages. When we express an idea, we have expressed ourselves; when we accept an idea, we have appropriated its sense and meaning. We have made what was foreign to us *our* own, and that is the essential task of hermeneutics. Because there are different degrees of understanding possible for us, there are several linguistic skills involved in their realization.

Currently, there exist three distinct, if alternative, definitions of hermeneutics: the first is based on the hermeneutic circle and pre-understanding, a tradition in hermeneutics; the second emphasizes dialogue between worlds that are incommensurable and thus require translation; and the third involves a hermeneutic in which understanding stands in a concrete and opaque relational totality that is not, in principle, a set of rules or propositions but, according to Palmer (in Shapiro & Sica, 1984), "human practices whose nature is never fully articulable in rational terms" (p. 85).

HISTORICAL BACKGROUND AND PHILOSOPHICAL ROOTS

From the very beginning, hermeneutics appears to have a double filiation, first with Romantic Philosophy and its appeal to the mind as "the creative unconscious at work in gifted individuals"; and secondly, with Critical Philosophy and its "wish to elaborate the universally valid rules of understanding" (Ricoeur, 1981, p. 46).

The hermeneutical problem of mediating the unfamiliar into understanding is as old as language itself. For example, it was posed in antiquity, according to Klemm (1983), in "the need to interpret messages of the gods, to deliver religious and moral commentary upon the Homeric epics," as well as to develop a "philosophical doctrine of rhetoric, and to achieve normative application" of authoritative texts (p. 18). Judaism met the hermeneutical problem in the task of interpreting the law through sacred scripture. Early in the Christian era (100–300 A.D.), the schools of Alexandria and Antioch were ranged against one another in a "hermeneutic" relationship. The former employed the allegorical, the latter the literal (or emphatic) method.

Historians of hermeneutics have argued that there are diverse sources reaching back to the traditions of Classical and Medieval rhetoric (see Table 1). The last great representative of this tradition was the prophetic thinker Vico. The tradition of practical philosophy that took shape as a result of Aristotle's reflections on "praxis" and "phronesis" is also prominent. The contributions of legal history and jurisprudence, the humanism of the Renaissance, as well as the post-Reformation discipline of biblical interpretation indicate that hermeneutics is closely intertwined with the entire history of humanistic studies (Bernstein, 1983).

Table 1
Intellectual Heritage of Hermeneutics

Greco-Latin Influence

Plato (427–347 B.C.) Dialogues, Conversations
Aristotle (384–322 B.C.) Praxis and Phronesis: Practical Philosophy
Alexandria and Antioch (100–300 A.D.) Hermeneutic: Allegorical and Literal Methods

First Scientific Hermeneutists

Flacius (1567)	Bengel (1740)	Wines (1822)
Glassius (1629)	Ernesto (1765)	

Classical and Medieval Rhetoric Influence

Vico (1700) Last representative: Anti-Cartesian

Modern Hermeneutics

Influences

Enlightenment
Romantic and
Critical Philosophy

Schleiermacher
Husserl
Historians: H. White
Q. Skinner, Collingwood
M. Hesse, C. Geertz

Kierkegaard
Husserl
Neitzsche

Frederick Schleiermacher (1768–1834)
Founder of Modern Hermeneutics
"Theory of the Art of Understanding"

Wilhem Dilthey (1833-1911)
Historical reason as method for
Geisteswissenschaften-Human sciences
"The Rise of Hermeneutics"

Martin Heidegger (1889-1976)
Existential Metaphysics
Phenomenological Hermeneutics
Being and Time

Hermeneutic Critiques

Influences

Plato
Aristotle
Hegel, Heidegger
Husserl
Nietzsche

Kant, Husserl
Marcel, Nabert
Structuralism
Critical Theory
Analytic Philosophy

Kant, Fichte
Marx, Dewey
Mead, J. H., Weber, M.
Durkheim, Parsons

Hans Georg Gadamer (1900-   )
Hermeneutic Circle, Dialogue and play
Fusion of hermeneutics and application
"Fusion of Horizons"
Truth and Method

Paul Ricoeur (1913-   )
Transforms Husserlian Phenomenology
Towards Hermeneutics
Theory of Interpretation: Distanciation
Hermeneutics and the Human Sciences

Hans Jurgen Habermas (1930-   )
"Performative Attitude: Theory of
Communicative Action and Rationality"
Knowledge and Human Interests

Interestingly, the New Encyclopedia of Philosophy (1957) names the first scientific hermeneutists as Flacius (1567) and Glassius (1629), who then were followed by Bengel (1740), Ernesto (1765), and Wines (1822). However, excerpts of the works of the following hermeneutists represent modern interpretations.

Frederick Schleiermacher (1768–1834)

In the nineteenth century, an appeal was made to hermeneutics to clarify what was distinctive about human science (Geisteswissenschaften) and natural science (Naturwissenschaften). Schleiermacher, founder of modern hermeneutics, was one of the first to argue for the general significance of hermeneutics and drew upon this tradition to meet the challenge of a then growing skepticism about religious understanding. According to Bornstein (1983), nineteenth-century hermeneutics developed as a reaction against "the intellectual imperialism of the growth of positivism, inductionism," and the type of scientism that claimed preeminence for the natural sciences in providing the model and standards for what is to count as genuine knowledge.

In the nineteenth century, hermeneutics was to form the basis of all human sciences. The old theological and literary discipline of hermeneutics had been transformed and broadened. The original pragmatic purpose of making literary texts more understandable was expanded to include, according to Gadamer (1975), "all that no longer expresses itself in and through its own world," such as art, history, culture, and language. Because human craft from the past is "estranged from its original meaning," it depends now, for its unlocking and communicating, "on the spirit that we, like the Greeks, name Hermes: the messenger of the Gods" (p. 146–147).[1]

Wilhem Dilthey (1833–1911)

Without much question, then, hermeneutics owes its central function within the human sciences to the development of an historical consciousness in which Dilthey plays a key role.

A follower of Schleiermacher, Dilthey extended the hermeneutic tradition to deal with two of the major intellectual problems of his age: the study of history and historical knowledge and, on the continent, the rival claims of those thinkers promoting the natural and human sciences. According to Dilthey, the primary task of hermeneutics was to determine the value of humanistic and historical knowledge in such a way that it would meet and challenge the prevailing view that only the natural sciences could provide "objective knowledge." Dilthey's task involved revealing the characteristic subject matter, aims, and methods of historical inquiry, specifically historical reason through philosophical hermeneutics (Bernstein, 1983). As will be seen, Dilthey's own reliance on natural science tenets for historical knowledge was criticized by later hermeneutists, especially Heidegger, Gadamer, and Ricoeur.[2]

Martin Heidegger (1889–1976)

In the twentieth century, primarily due to the Phenomenological Movement, in particular, Heidegger's *Being and Time* (1962), hermeneutics has moved into a position central to European philosophy. Heidegger extended the nature of hermeneutics from an epistemological endeavor to a claim for ontological significance and universality. Rather than a subdiscipline of humanistic studies or as the method of Geisteswissenschaften (human sciences), hermeneutics was viewed as pertaining to questions concerning "what human beings are" (in Bernstein, 1983, p. 113). In fact, Heidegger (in Ricoeur, 1981) did not conceive of understanding as a way of knowing but as a "mode of being," as a fundamental characteristic of our "being-in-the-world" (p. 20).[3]

Hans Georg Gadamer (1900–   )

Gadamer, as one of the preeminent hermeneutists of the German Romantic tradition, sought to answer questions related to practical philosophy. His critique of hermeneutics is highly regarded, along with those of Ricoeur and Habermas, in Anglo-American Philosophy, especially since 1970.

Gadamer addresses the implications and significance of hermeneutics for understanding the limits and role of the social and political disciplines.[4] His book, *Truth and Method*, is, according to Bernstein (1983), one of the "most comprehensive and subtle statements of the meaning and scope of hermeneutics of this century" (p. 34).

Because the primary focus of Gadamer's efforts is on hermeneutic experience, works of art, the understanding and interpretation of literary texts, and the study of history all come into play. However, unlike Heidegger, his teacher, who adopted a radical style of thinking by which to pursue ultimate questions, Gadamer (1975) poses more humble questions with a sense toward "what is feasible, possible, correct, or here and now" (p. xxv).[5]

Finally, Gadamer's work culminates in a theory of historical consciousness as the foundation of the human sciences, which will be explained in more detail later on.[6] A significant task in this effort was Gadamer's move to legitimize the hermeneutic circle of understanding, a primary hermeneutic process, through explication of the notions of dialogue and conversation.

For example, in contrast to Dilthey, Gadamer is emphatically opposed to the distancing of the interpreter advocated by the natural sciences to achieve objective knowledge. Gadamer argues that such distancing, even if it were possible, is destructive to the very nature of belonging, an ontological given between interpreter and the world in dialogue. Unfortunately, Gadamer is not able to close the gulf created between explanation (distanciation of the sciences) and understanding (belongingness of hermeneutics) as he interprets them. However, Gadamer is acknowledged by Habermas (1971) to have achieved a fusion of hermeneutics and application in praxis. And, according to Bernstein (1983), this becomes the most central theme in Gadamer's analysis of philosophic hermeneutics.[7]

Appropriately, then, Gadamer's principal contribution to the hermeneutic tradition is his concept of "effective-historical consciousness." He asserts that a relation of affinity and a sense of belongingness exists between us and an alien text or tradition that we seek to understand. As Gadamer sees it (in Bernstein, 1983), "We belong to a tradition before it belongs to us" (p. 142). Therefore, the task Gadamer sets before philosophic hermeneutics is to stand in "effective-historical consciousness"; that is, to feel this belongingness, and in this dialogue between self and historical horizon mediated through language, to enlarge and deepen both. Rather than a specific procedure, a fusion of horizons is thus made possible through the universal characteristic of "linguisticality"; a concept that Gadamer develops into a theory of the universality of language. Without such a theory, a fusion of horizons could not otherwise be achieved. According to Gadamer, being itself is "housed within" languages. Therefore, to fuse the past and present, as Bleicher (1980) explains it, one asks a question of the text and the text provides an answer through philosophical reflection on this type of dialogic conversation.

Paul Ricoeur (1913–   )[8]

As previously stated, neither Heidegger nor Gadamer were able to reconcile the philosophical gulf between the process of explanation and understanding. Ricoeur's greatest contribution to hermeneutics, however, is a theory of interpretation which ultimately answers this problem.

It is, in fact, Ricoeur's (1981) concept of "distanciation" that offers a means toward the creation of the theory mentioned above. Ricoeur suggests that the initial hermeneutical question be such that "a certain dialectic between the experience of belonging and alienating distanciation becomes the mainspring, the key to the inner life of hermeneutics" (p. 90).

By the process of distanciation (refer to the section on Research Processes for further elaboration), the text is treated as an autonomous discourse and focal point of interpretation. The semantic autonomy of the text becomes the very condition of historical understanding of the present in light of the past. In terms of human science, this was a remarkable breakthrough.[9]

Hans Jurgen Habermas (1930–   )

Habermas (1971) is our most recent and significant critical hermeneutist. His work focuses on "communicative action," which he defines as an interaction of humans which leads to understanding; his approach is a critical reconstructive analysis. To his credit, Habermas recognized within Gadamer's *Truth and Method* that a link was made between hermeneutical understanding and the transcendental necessity of articulating an "action-oriented self-understanding" (Bernstein, 1983). This insight led Habermas further to see hermeneutics not only as helpful in highlighting the limitations of positivists' modes of thought but also to highlighting the hermeneutical dimension essential to all social knowledge. Thus, hermeneutics would be helpful in answering his major question, which concerns a foundation for a critical theory of society.[10] However, in time Habermas realized the need to elaborate a comprehensive "theory of rationality" to address normative action.[11]

While Gadamer's contributions and focus were on understanding "understanding" itself, Habermas' contribution and focus were on understanding as it shapes the foundation of practical discourse and its role in redeeming normative validity or rightness for human action (Klemm, 1983).

In addition, the rationality Habermas proposes is eventually meant to address two types of human action: (1) purposive-rational actions (also known as "technical") and (2) communicative action (also known as "praxis"). His rationality is not meant to provide a blueprint for action but rather a comprehensive theory for action. As an ontological foundation of discourse, understanding for Habermas has become the center of both types of action, the validity of which is to be decided by the participants in the discourse.

Habermas is one of the most complex yet promising figures for twenty-first century hermeneutics and human science. He provides a method of reconstructive analysis for human science and certainly provides a philosophical critique of hermeneutics that has *heuristic* (life learning) value for a practice discipline with ethical dimensions, such as nursing.

This brief, historical introduction to the philosophical roots and epistemological assumptions of hermeneutic tradition will continue below in the discussion on researcher preparation and the research processes.

PREPARATION AND CHARACTERISTICS OF THE HERMENEUTIC INTERPRETER

Many suggestions have been made for the preparation and necessary characteristics of the hermeneutic interpreter. This section draws upon rich sources of hermeneutic wisdom and provides a broad range of talents which are in need of development.

The Art of Understanding the Author of the Text

The art of interpretation is a craft rather than a mechanistic operation. To place technical approaches in proper perspective, Schleiermacher (1977) said that "comparison" of texts to texts and authors to authors is important but, in itself, is an insufficient tool for understanding. He insisted that an interpreter needs some talent for "feeling" or "divining" how language as a living, organic power has affected the fabric of thought and the mode of presentation. Also necessary is some insight into the kind of person who writes in order to describe how "qualities unique to the author shaped the production . . . "(p. 5).

If the task of the interpreter is to understand the author of the text, which is one approach common to theological hermenuetics described by Schleiermacher, then part of the interpreter's preparation is to learn about the author's life. Yet Schleiermacher (1977) also recognized that it is in "understanding the person's statement that the interpreter comes to learn about the one who makes them" (p. 5).

In addition, it is helpful for the interpreter to act like an artisan between the life of the languaged text and the life of the author; that is, in a back and forth motion, tacking like a sailor does a boat, toward the goal of understanding. Quite literally, the interpreter is to be suspended between the universal and particular aspects of the text. According to Schleiermacher (1977), this hermeneutic posture requires "agility, an ability to weave from grammatical to psychological side and from comparative to divinatory method" (p. 6). Ultimately, interpretation is always open to revision and supplementation. Therefore, it is always an approximation and never perfect or complete.

Skills of Exegeses

Additional linguistic skills for the interpreter in the early nineteenth century are relevant for use today. Schleiermacher (1977) includes the use of parallel passages; the notion of *accommodation*, of a passage to something originally not intended on the grounds of resemblance or analogy; the difference between literal and figurative meaning; and the propriety of stressing or discounting certain terms.

However, it is important while in the midst of the detail of interpretation, to keep clearly in view that the ultimate goal for Schleiermacher was to understand fully the unique messages that formed New Testament texts. To accomplish such an understanding, the hermeneutic process brought together the technical, psychological, and grammatical aspects of language, which required then as now a highly refined and subtle expertise.

Characteristics of the Interpreter

Charles Taylor (1979) has defended the hermeneutic circle as an eminently helpful interpretive method in the human sciences in the twentieth century. Drawing upon ideas from Aristotle, Taylor (in Rabinow & Sullivan, 1979) suggests the following characteristics for the successful prosecution of heremeneutics: "A high degree of self-knowledge and a freedom from illusion, in the sense of error which is rooted and expressed in one's way of life" (p. 71).

Taylor believes that our incapacity to understand is rooted in our own self-definitions; hence, in what we are. The interpreter must also have the insight, imagination, openness, and patience to acquire the art of understanding—an art achieved through practice. There is no determinate method for acquiring or pursuing this art, in the sense of explicit rules that are to be followed; however, there are heuristic guides that hermeneutists recommend.

Rules of Interpretation

Paul Ricoeur (1981) presents two views on the rules of interpretation that are common threads throughout the hermeneutic tradition. One set of rules is animated by faith and sympathy; the other by an attitude of suspicion and doubt. The first attitude is reflected in the hermeneutics of theological inquiry which characterizes an interpreter's willingness to listen to the world in the given text and respect the symbols as revelations of the sacred. Hermeneutics is construed as the restoration of a meaning addressed to the interpreter in the form of a message regardless of the era in which he or she lives.

In contrast, another type of hermeneutic is regarded as a demystification of a meaning presented to the interpreter in the form of a disguise. Ricoeur (1981) suggests that Marx, Neitzsche, and Freud practiced the latter type of hermeneutic. Skepticism towards the given and distrust of the symbol as a "dissimulation of the real" (p. 6) are characteristic of this view. The contents of consciousness expressed in language are regarded to be in some sense false. However, according to Ricoeur, all three— Marx, Nietzsche, and Freud—aimed to transcend this falsity through a reductive interpretation and critique.

Ricoeur (1981) also offers us a bit of wisdom by combining these two attitudes and saying, "as a reader, I find myself only by losing myself" (p. 144). He reminds would-be interpreters that ultimately to understand is to understand "oneself in front of the text" (p. 143) instead of hidden within the text. It is not a question of imposing upon the text our finite capacity of understanding, but of exposing ourselves to the text and receiving from it an enlarged self.

Distanciation Versus Belonging: The Gadamer Debate

Gadamer (in Ricoeur, 1981) argued that the methodology of the natural sciences implies a "distancing" which, in turn, expresses the "destruction of the primordial relation of belonging without which there would be no relation to the historical as such" (p. 60). The debate between alienating distanciation and the experience of belonging is pursued by Gadamer throughout the three spheres in which he divides the hermeneutical experience: (1) The esthetic sphere, in which taste is the judgment; (2) the historical sphere, which refers to the traditions which precede us; and (3) the language sphere, which includes the other two spheres as well as the co-belonging to tradition or the things "great voices have said" (p. 60). In all three spheres, Gadamer argues against distanciation as a means toward objectivity. In contrast, his position on belonging through the use of language ultimately bridges the past and present horizons.

Attitudes for Interpreter Preparation

Currently, the attitudes of distancing and belonging are themes which have relevance to the dialectic being played out between critical and feminist theory towards a true emancipation of scholarship in the human sciences (Benhabib & Cornell, 1987) as well as practice in the world of nursing (Fiorenza, 1984; Thompson, 1987; Allen, 1987). Underlying this dialectic are qualitative and quantitative distinctions. On the side of qualitative criteria, Gadamer (in Bernstein 1983) suggests for interpreter preparation that

> we must learn the art of being responsive to works of art, texts, and traditions (other persons or forms of life) that we are trying to understand. We must participate in or share them, listen to them, open ourselves to what they are saying and to the claims to truth that they make upon us. (p. 137)

Gadamer further believes that we can accomplish this type of understanding only because of the forestructures (language and culture) and prejudgments (experience, norms, and mores of our lives) that are constitutive of our being. This position exemplifies animation by Gadamer from a hermeneutic attitude of "faith or sympathy" rather than from one of "suspicion" as a starting point for the interpreter.

The Performative Attitude

In contrast, quantitative criteria for distancing can be identified in Habermas (1971), who superficially exemplifies the hermeneutic attitude of "suspicion and doubt" as a starting point but actually blends the two attitudes of distancing and belonging in a new synthesis.

Habermas (in Bernstein, 1983) suggests that if we want to describe other forms of life or earlier stages of our own social development, then we can only do this by "adopting the performative attitude"; that is, the attitude of "one who participates in a process of mutual understanding" (p. 182). In other words, Habermas proposes a critical approach to understanding but suggests it be introduced before assimilating the experience at hand. That is, belonging to a world with other persons with whom we must participate in coming to know it actively also is a critical process rather than one merely of "faith or sympathy." This attitude will be described further in the section on research processes.

Experience-Near and Experience-Distant Perspective

Clifford Geertz (1976, 1979), an anthropologist who uses hermeneutics, provides further insight on interpreter preparation. Anthropologists ask the question: "How is anthropological knowledge of the way natives think, feel, and perceive possible?" Geertz (in Bernstein, 1983) introduces the distinction between "experience-near and experience-distant" and suggests that the best solution is to focus on "how anthropological analysis is to be conducted and its results framed, rather than what psychic constitution anthropologists need to have" (p. 94). He does acknowledge that anthropologists need to be sensitive and imaginative, need to listen carefully and to see accurately, but criticizes the bias that what is special about the anthropologist is that he or she can achieve "some sort of psychic unity with the people of interest" (p. 94). Geertz (1976) continues:

> What is required of the anthropologist is close attention to searching out and analyzing the symbolic forms, words, images, institutions, behaviors–in terms of which people actually represent themselves to themselves and to one another. (p. 228)

In summary, the recommended preparation of a researcher in the hermeneutical method would include a thorough reading of the historical background, philosophical roots and assumptions of the hermeneutical tradition, and, second, a contrast and comparison of various perspectives on hermeneutic techniques of analysis, reconstruction, and artistries for achieving understanding.

The selection of hermeneutical approaches will depend upon the kind of text to be interpreted (language, art, historico-cultural structures, or meaningful human actions) and will be influenced by the idea animating the researcher.

Hermeneutical strategies and attitudes can enhance high level scholarship in graduate programs of nursing. These include sympathetic and critical appraisal, use of the hermeneutic circle of understanding, distanciation, belonging, appropriation, performative attitude, reflection, linguistic interpretive skills, and structural analysis, to name a few primary skills of scholarship.

THE RESEARCH PROCESS

Hermeneutists have made significant strides toward increased understanding of texts, narrowly and broadly conceived. Key processes are suggested in their works and are helpful within the context of the author's design and purpose.

The initial two primary processes are taken from Schleiermacher (1977). The first provides a framework designated as the grammatical and technical interpretation of biblical texts; the second provides a description of the hermeneutic circle and its changing role in the art of understanding.

First, it is important to note that in Schleiermacher's (1977) earlier work on "language as process" he held the notion that language and thought were identical. Thus, the intention of the author was accessible through written discourse. Later, Schleiermacher conceived of thought as a purely ideal reality that, by necessity, was modified when rendered in the form of empirical language. Therefore, if the text as written no longer represented the intention of the author as a pure ideal, then another question could be raised: what claim did historical sources hold on life.

The Theory of the Art of Understanding

To know modern hermeneutics is to first know Schleiermacher (1977) and then the variations introduced by hermeneutists thereafter. Schleiermacher answered the above question with the notion of shared language. For example, a speaker stands under the power of language, its conventions and rules, which allow one to speak while still conditioning one's pattern of thought. Yet, the message one thinks and articulates is one's own. If this is so, two sides of language exist and need to be investigated for understanding. Schleiermacher developed a theory of "the art of understanding" from this assumption. It is outlined below in the form of a heuristic guide for research design and process.

Outline of Schleiermacher's Methods. Central to Schleiermacher's (1977) theory is that linguistic expression (text and living speech) has a twofold reference: (1) "to the objective meaning in the context of the entire language, and (2) to the specific thought in the entire life of the speaker or author" (p. 97–98). According to Klemm (1981), this combination of elements in the linguistic expression requires in turn the combination of two methods of intrepretation: (1) "grammatical interpretation," which focuses on the common language itself in order to grasp the linguistic usage of the author so that the text may be placed in its linguistic contexts, and (2) "technical or psychological interpretation" (p. 21), which aims to gain full understanding of the author's individual stylistic use of language to express his or her experience and thought.

Together, these two methods of interpretation express the hermeneutic circle. In *grammatical interpretation*, the interpreter endeavors to reproduce the "sphere of language" shared by the author and the original audience. In this broader linguistic context, then, each word, sentence, section, and work is placed as it belongs to the whole.

In *technical-psychological interpretation*, the author's command of the language as style comes forward. The interpreter penetrates the peculiar message of a work by way of the author's distinctive use of language. Within this approach, the interpreter examines the form and organization used by the author and also considers the initial decision or idea which impels the author to communicate. Thus, the form and organization is in dialectic with the author's impelling motive, which carries the composition to its completion.

Though presented separately, the two methods of interpretation are meant to be inseparable and interrelated. According to Schleiermacher (1977), the "deft interplay" of the two produce the constant revisions characteristic of this linguistic art.

An "expression" is considered by Schleiermacher, then, to be a thought that has been concretized from an infinite number of possibilities which refer to a series of linguistic contexts, such as: words in sentences, sentences in a paragraph, paragraphs within a work, etc. In addition, an expression is the product of free, individual, and artistic thinking which externalizes itself in a given language. Ultimately, for Schleiermacher (1977), "the meaning of the expression can only be approximated in understanding by feeling" (p. 77), since what is most important about the expression as an esthetic construct is the original experience behind the thought that is expressed.

Again, for Schleiermacher (1977), the aim in understanding a written expression from a previous time is to "understand the text at first as well as and then even better than its author" (p. 112). This is to be achieved by creatively coordinating the grammatical and technical-psychological methods in such a way as to make conscious much of what the author could not have known. As interpreted by Klemm (1983):

> Each method is pursued dialectally along the hermeneutic circle so that meaning is secured with increasing depth and precision by referring it from part to whole, expressions to context, and back again from whole to part. (p. 21)

Schleiermacher (1977) provides the interpreter with two additional canons to govern the grammatical interpretation. These canons define the "circle" in language and state that:

1. Meanings are to be determined in their individuality through feeling the sense of word-meanings current at the time the author wrote.

2. Each passage must be considered as the peculiar shaping of a simple meaning through the reciprocal relations between it and the context of the work.

Thus, grammatical interpretation presupposes knowing the language as the author knew it in his or her time in history. This prepares the way for an intuitive grasp of the author as a person.

The Divinatory and Comparative Methods. For Schleiermacher (1977), the goal in technical-psychological interpretation is to uncover the theme of the works as the impelling motive behind the author's expressions. Two more methods are used for this purpose, however: (1) In the "divinatory" method or "feeling" method, the interpreter is to attune to the author intuitively through his or her language as a living, organic power which has affected the fabric of thought and the mode of presentation. The author as an individual comes forth. (2) The comparative method subsumes the author's work under archetypes of language and form that are distinct or similar in trait to the work being interpreted. Interpretation of a work is completed, therefore, when the results of grammatical interpretation agree with the results of technical-psychological interpretation.[12]

Hermeneutic Circle

The second major insight of Schleiermacher is the hermeneutic circle. The metaphor of a circle is most apt for the dynamic movement within hermeneutics. According to Schleiermacher (1977), the hermeneutic circle is a logical vexing proposition: "The whole is understood from its parts and the parts from the whole and means that interpretation is at the base of a referential procedure" (p. 5–6). This proposition is applied at every crucial point of Schleiermacher's theory for the art of understanding although the term itself had not yet been coined. It is the motion in hermeneutics which makes it an art.

The hermeneutic circle is most clearly applied to the written text. Just as each word is determined by its position in the sentence (subject, predicate, object) so each passage and section of a work is to be read in light of the whole. Yet each sentence yields its meaning from the words it contains, and the work as a whole is understood by what each of its various parts presents. More comprehensively, each work is to be seen in relation to the totality of language by reference to what is spoken and written. Language carries the tradition, culture and mores of a people. It provides the structure for expression that reflects the past, present and future (tense), the agent of action (first, second or third person) as well as the context (conditional phrases) and particular and universal characteristics (modifiers). Language is a powerful entity in itself and is the most unique of human characteristics.

Difference and Distance between Persons in Conversation. Hermeneutics, which is based on the phenomenon of understanding, acknowledges an initial difference and distance between persons in a conversation; one wishes to communicate, and the other wishes to understand. Thus, the dance or interplay begins. The difference between players is not absolute, however, for it is, according to Schleiermacher (1977), "mitigated by a shared language and a common humanity. Secured upon these two rocks, hermeneutics bridges the distance between partners in conversations" (p. 13).

Schleiermacher's (1977) theory also reflects a new relationship to history and historical sources. Again, hermeneutics spans the distance between persons, author, and reader, but "these persons are now separated by the ages, by altered ways of viewing and relating to the world, and by changing patterns of thought" (p. 13). For example, the historical text is no longer addressed directly to the present interpreter, but to an original audience. Thus, the present interpreter is to understand that original communication in terms of its historical context.

An awareness that the present interpreter is disadvantaged by loss of an immediate understanding and sense of an immediate applicability of the past for the present was seen by Kimmerle as critical to Schleiermacher (1977). The historical contents must be grasped first in terms of their historical context. Understanding remains the central concern of hermeneutics and the art of understanding (the hermeneutic circle) is the lasting contribution of Schleiermacher to the history of hermeneutic theory.

Dilthey and Historical Applications of the Hermeneutic Circle

Dilthey takes Schleiermacher's hermeneutic circle of understanding and uses it as the necessary condition for the possibility of understanding historical expressions. Dilthey extends the hermeneutic circle to dialogue between individual lived experience and the realm of historical expressions. The latter are always expressions of life, such as a common heritage of language, law, morals, art, and culture. In his *Der Aufbau* (1927), Dilthey emphasized that expression always comes from an irreducible individual: as such, expression refers to the interconnectedness of everything in life and specifically from which it arose. Klemm (1983) further explains that written expressions are transparent to the individual author, and their intended meanings refer to interconnecting cultural contexts.[13]

According to Klemm (1983), who examined the original writings of Dilthey, the hermeneutic circle is comprised of the interplay between ideal meanings expressed in signs and the flux of life in things, events, processes, and states of affairs. Thus, acquaintance with the common cultural world is necessary for the sophisticated understanding of individual texts. Further, expertise in the human and moral sciences enables higher levels of understanding but Dilthey also recognized that prior to all of this understanding is a "doxic" (or fundamental) prereflective lived experience of the world out of which the art of understanding is constituted.

Dilthey builds upon Husserl's notion of inner-time consciousness (intentionality), which reflects the convergance of the past, future, and the present. For example, the art of understanding is explained, first, in the present, as an "empathic transposition of the self into the other self" (in Klemm, 1983, p. 25). The past is relived through this empathic transposition and the future is presented through a reconstruction of the past (historical experience).

Dilthey gives major emphasis to "self-recognition" within the development of historical experience for an individual. In other words, self-recognition is self-knowledge derived from experience of the world in the present which then becomes part of the past to be recalled again and again.

Heidegger's Ontological Use of the Hermeneutic Circle. Heidegger (1962) transformed the meaning, scope, and significance of the hermeneutic circle. One important distinction made by Heidegger within the circle of understanding is the priority given to "reference" (objectivity of being-world) over "sense" (subjectivity of author or interpreter). As interpreted by Klemm (1983), Heidegger does not refer to problems addressed by either Schleiermacher or Dilthey but rather begins with a focus on hermeneutics as "interpretation of human being" (p. 26). This is an ontological turn within the tradition of hermeneutics based on Heidegger's existential and speculative philosophical background. Heidegger does not focus on interpretation of texts but on "the interpretation in existential concepts of the understanding of being that *Dasein* has already laid out publicly in its world through its discourse" (p. 27). (*Dasein* is a German expression for "our humanness or very being.") Heidegger's goal is to "think the meaning of being by way of hermeneutics"; he begins with *Dasein* as the place where being is manifest and uses hermeneutics to interpret *Dasein* for its meaning. One of his basic assumptions is that an obscurity and forgetfulness surround the meaning of being, even though it is the most fundamental word and thought in the language. Heidegger contends that we possess an implicit (pre-ontological) understanding of the meaning of being, but we lack an explicit concept of it.[14]

The hermeneutic circle is extended by Heidegger to the ontological expression of *Dasein* itself as an understanding, caring mode of being.[15] The goal of Heidegger is to provide the foundation of "being as being" to undergird an understanding of all knowledge.[16]

Gadamer's Dialogic Play as Hermeneutic Circle

One of Gadamer's (1975a) tasks was to legitimize the hermeneutic circle of understanding, and he chose to do so through an explication of the notion of dialogue, conversation, and freedom in his book *Truth and Method*. As interpreted by Bernstein (1983), "play" is the "clue to ontological explanation illustrating the nature of dialogue" (p. 161). Gadamer (1975) clarifies this notion further:

> When one enters into a dialogue with another person and then is carried further by the dialogue, it is no longer the will of the individual person, holding itself back or exposing itself, that is determinative. Rather, the law of the subject matter [die sache] is at issue in the dialogue and elicits statements and counter statements, and in the end plays them into each other. (p. 347)

Thus, conversation between two persons is a process whereby each player in the dialogue is open to the other and accepts the other's point of view for what it is. Then, in getting inside the other to such an extent, one can come to understand what the other says. Gadamer (1975) does not say the end result of dialogue is coming to understand a particular individual. Rather, agreement is the important benefit of dialogue. As he says: "The thing that has to be grasped is the objective rightness or otherwise of his opinion, so that they can agree with each other on the subject" (p. 347).

Gadamer, like Heidegger, emphasizes the importance of the ontological, existential side of dialogue as the source of objective truth which can be agreed upon; the subject matter (content) guides the movement of the dialogue. However, elsewhere Gadamer emphasizes the method (hermeneutic experience) in saying that the centrality of self-knowledge [die Sache selbst] guides us founded upon "recognition" of ourselves as like and different from the other in dialectical encounter with the other.[17]

Gadamer is less driven toward absolute truth than he is to understand understanding itself as it pertains to works of art, literary texts, and history. It is important to remember that Gadamer lived before the post-empiricist period in science, so he retains a positivist view of science and objectivity even in his discussion of play and dialogue.

Place of Prejudice and Prejudgments in Understanding. Gadamer (1979) transforms the hermeneutic circle in a way that clarifies the place of prejudice and prejudgments in understanding. As indicated, attention is given to the "things themselves" (p. 151), so they can speak to us; however, as Bernstein (1983) puts it, we do not do this by "bracketing or forgetting all our prejudgments and prejudices" (p. 138).

The key lies in the interplay of prejudgments and prejudices which enables us to understand the "things themselves" (Gadamer, 1979, p. 152). These are called by Heidegger as well as Gadamer the forestructures of the interpreter or the horizon. The difference between prejudices that blind us from the meaning and truth of what we want to understand and those that enable us to understand is made clear by our opening ourselves to the "newness" of what is handed down to us, and through the play between our forestructures and the "things themselves." As a result, a "fusion of horizons" is effected to enlarge understanding for the reader.

Understanding and interpretation are not different but are the same for Gadamer. Thus, the process of understanding can never (ontologically) achieve finality because, as such, we are always interpreting in light of our anticipatory prejudgments and prejudices which are themselves always changing in the course of history. Meaning for Gadamer (1975a), therefore, is always "coming into being" (p. 257) through the happening of understanding.

The Understanding-Appropriation Process. The understanding-appropriation process is made possible through the linguistic nature of human beings. The event of appropriation happens only if the text is permitted to speak into the openness of the reader's linguistic world. For Gadamer (1975a), the horizons come from the author's linguistic world of tradition and that of the reader, and together they are enlarged and deepened into understanding.[18]

Underlying the possibility of appropriation is the "belongingness to the traditions" that every interpreter has. According to Klemm (1987), often the tradition is appropriated passively. However, Gadamer (1976) suggests that if newness is to be concretized by the event of appropriation, the reader must be capable of listening, and of being "negative to his or her immediate and surface experience" (p. 450). Thus, the reader is to disengage his or her preconceptions by allowing the ontological world to open to them. Ricoeur develops the process of understanding-appropriation further in his theory of interpretation as distanciation.

Application of Hermeneutics to Praxis. Gadamer's primary success in philosophy was to fuse hermeneutics and its applications. According to Bernstein (1983), the type of knowledge and truth hermeneutics yields is practical knowledge and truth that shapes our "praxis" (p. 150). Gadamer states that the chief task of philosophic hermeneutics is to "correct the peculiar falsehood of modern consciousness" and "to defend practical and political reason against the domination of technology based on science" (p. 150).

Again, the primordial mode of being is understanding itself; and language is not simply a tool for understanding but is the medium in which self-knowledge comes into being and continues to unfold. Gadamer's positions in hermeneutics have had tremendous appeal partially because of the comprehensiveness of his scholarship and its relevance to practical concerns and moral implications.

Ricoeur's Concept of Text: Naive Reading to Structural Analysis

Reading as the recovery of meaning is the theme of Ricoeur's works. He provides a classification of written texts which require a variety of hermeneutic procedures for understanding their meaning. The beginning place is that of reading the descriptive text and gleaning the apparent single or literal meaning. No sophisticated procedures are necessary but a naive reading will suffice at this level.

The second kind of text in Ricoeur's scheme consists of the literary or poetic texts that, defined by their double meaning, require interpretive effort. For Ricoeur, the hermeneutic problem is between "sense" and "event" in discourse. Thus, the dialogue must be located in discourse. In literary or poetic texts, a second and indirect sense is presented and points to a second and indirect reference. The hermeneutic process requires adding to these the initial literal and direct sense-referent configuration. Literary texts play on the figurative and suggestive power of language to express "modes of being in the world." Cosmic and psychic symbols are created by the imagination and point to referents in a possible or suggested world, but must also point to the literal referent of the perceptual world. This is so because the figurative sense is present only as a suggestion made by the literal sense. For example, the unicorn is the figurative sense of an object that looks like a horse with one horn extending from its forehead. Unicorn is a suggestion that arises from the literal sense that the object is not simply a horse but something other. It requires imagination and freedom to play with possible worlds to create the unicorn that has no natural reference in the actual world.[19]

Structural Analysis: Deliberate Processing of Distanciation.[20] After a naive reading of the text for surface meaning, structural analysis of the text, as reconstructed by Ricouer (1981), directs the interpreter to read the text from a critical stance for depth, semantic sense, and reference rather than for syntactical sense alone. In Ricoeur's hermeneutics, "reflection" is a deliberate interpretive critique to overcome immediate naive misunderstandings of a text.[21]

Ricoeur's Hermeneutic Theory of Interpretation-Distanciation. The written discourse defines the object domain of hermeneutics as the text. Thus, the *concept of text* as written discourse becomes the beginning place for hermeneutics. Ricoeur also emphasizes the concept of distanciation. The objective meaning of a text, thereby, is something other than the subjective intentions of its author. The problem of right understanding can no longer be solved by a simple return to the alleged intention of the author. The meaning of a text has to be guessed or construed as a whole. If more than one meaning results, Ricoeur (1981) recommends that the conflict be subjected to a process of argumentation in which the author has no privileged role. Since the text is removed from its original audience, two possible attitudes can be taken by the interpreter: (1) the attitude of epoché in which judgment is suspended about the referential dimension of the text, leaving a worldless and self-enclosed entity, or (2) the attitude of seeking to unfold the non-ostensive or less obvious references of the text, that is, a structuralist approach in which internal language relations explain the text. In Ricoeur's reconstruction, the interpreter is to seek something in *front* of the text—not something hidden behind or of the internal constitution of text—but that which indicates a possible world. Here one moves from "sense" of text to its "reference," "from that which it says to that which it says it is about" (p. 161).[22]

Distanciation criteria include four distinct types which can be identified in written expression. Ricoeur (1981) presents them as the conditions for the possibility of interpreting any written text objectively. In summary, four forms of distanciation can be recognized in the following examples:

1. Meaning that is inscribed in writing by virtue of the intentional externalization of the speech act.
2. Relation between inscribed expression and original speaker. What the text signifies no longer coincides with what the author meant.
3. Discrepancy between the inscribed expressions and the original audience. Text decontextualizes itself from its social and historical conditions of production, opening itself to unlimited readings.
4. Emancipations of the text from the limits of ostensive (internal) reference. A shared reality no longer exists as it did in speaking to one who is present. Thus, the referential dimension is of a different order from that of speech, which is unfolded in the process of interpretation (p. 13).

Distanciation or objectification of language is the counterpart of two other essential processes in Ricoeur's (1981) theory of interpretation: first, *belonging* to a history and culture and, second, *appropriation*, which is the making familiar of what was foreign. As described above, a new meaning is achieved by linking these two processes by a distanciation strategy such as structural analysis.

Appropriation Process. The process of interpretation culminates in an act of appropriation which forms the concluding counterpart of distanciation for Ricoeur (1981). To appropriate means to make one's own "what was initially alien" (p. 18). The act of appropriation does not seek to rejoin the original intentions of the author but rather to *expand the conscious horizons of the reader by actualizing the meaning of the text*; it is bound to the revelatory power of the text, to its power to *disclose a possible world*. Thus, Ricoeur leads us to a *concrete ontology in which what was possible becomes an actualized meaning of the text.*

For Ricoeur, the time of criticism and restoration in hermeneutics occurs at the same time. In other words, the criticism is no longer reductive but restorative. According to Klemm (1983), a common conviction among Schleiermacher, Dilthey, and Ricoeur is that by "interpreting . . . we can 'hear' again" in spite of the fact that "immediate belief" has been lost forever through critique. Invariably, for them, the common aim of hermeneutics is to restore a "mediated immediacy of meaning" by which the reader "can be called again" (p. 20).

Extension of Ricoeur's Theory to Other Domains. It is possible to regard *human action* as text, insofar as it may be objectified in a way that embodies the four forms of distanciation described above, that is, the event of doing is eclipsed by the significance of what is done. Ricoeur's (1981) criteria state: (1) An action is a meaningful entity which must be construed as a whole. (2) A conflict of interpretation can only be resolved by a process of argumentation and debate. The intentions of the agent may be relevant but are not decisive. (3) Structural analysis can be transposed into the social sphere and can provide an explanatory moment which mediates a depth interpretation of action.

Ricoeur's (1981) hermeneutics holds the basic assumption that human action displays a sense as well as a reference; it possesses an internal structure as well as projecting a possible world, "a potential mode of human existence which can be unfolded through the process of interpretation" (p. 16). Action itself is the referent of many texts.

Extension to History. As mentioned earlier, distanciation is the counterpart of belonging. Both historical experience and writing are instances of distanciation; each once belonged to, but now are distanced from, their source. Bernstein (1983) states: "By recognizing the values of the past only through their differences from those of the present, history opens up the real towards the possible" (p. 17). Thus, the past can mirror to us what is desirable and undesirable in the present and impel us to take action and to create the kind of world that is desirable.

Extension to Socio-Historical World. According to Bernstein (1983), hermeneutical distanciation, under the influence of the French philosopher Jean Nabert, gave the process of reflection a new meaning. Instead of a process of epistemological justification of knowledge, Nabert conceives reflection as "the recovery of the effort to exist and the desire to be" (p. 17). Existential attitudes and efforts are the focus of reflection. These efforts cannot be grasped immediately in an act of intellectual intuition and can only be glimpsed through the mirror of the objects and acts, the symbols and signs, wherein they are disclosed. "Hence," according to Ricoeur (1981), "reflections must become interpretation because I cannot grasp the act of existing except in signs scattered in the world" (p. 17). Reflection is by definition self-reflection, and thus raises the question of what the self might signify. But it is Habermas (1971) who restores a central role to "the self" in his theory of hermeneutics.

Critical Hermeneutics: Habermas

Habermas' (1971) reconstructive analysis of hermeneutics seeks to eluci-date universal conditions and rules that are implicit in linguistic compe-tence and in cognitive moral development. Habermas' purpose is to overcome the distinction between a posteriori (experiential) and a priori (nonexperiential) knowledge made by Kant. For him, hermeneutics is not a transcendental theory but rather an empirical, scientific theory. As interpreted by Bernstein (1983), Habermas' goal is to outline a re-search program for a universal pragmatics that aspires to identify and reconstruct the universal conditions of possible understanding.

Habermas' Theory of Communicative Action and Rationality. Communicative action is a social interaction oriented toward understanding. It is distinct from non-social instrumental action and social strategic action, both of which are oriented toward "success." Communicative action exhibited in speech acts is the focus of Habermas' hermeneutics. The goal is to come to an understanding to bring about an *agreement* that terminates in the intersubjective mutuality of reciprocal understanding, shared knowledge, mutual trust, and accord with one another. Habermas' terms of agreement can be recognized by validity claims which include the following characteristics: (1) comprehensibility, (2) truth, (3) truthful-ness, and (4) rightness.

This critical hermeneutic method is discourse and consists in elucida-tion and argumentation in which immediate action is suspended and participants seek to redeem the validity claims that have been challenged. These are never ideal; even some "breaks" in communication are resolved by means of a variety of nondiscursive strategies.

The above four types of validity claims pose the following guidelines:

1. If what is said is not heard as intelligible or comprehensible, then seek mutual agreement to help make utterances comprehensible.

2. If comprehensible, then is it true? Then theoretical discourse is used to ascertain the truth of *statements made* or *implied*.

3. If you suspect lying or deceit, then determine the truthfulness of what is *said* in the actual statements.

4. Is it appropriate or right; what is the implied claim to normative validity? This requires a *practical* discourse with the other that will redeem the normative validity claim of the action in question.

ISSUES OF GENERALIZABILITY, VALIDITY, AND RELIABILITY

These three criteria of scientific knowledge can be subsumed under the hermeneutic requirement for "adequacy of interpretation." Taylor (in Bernstein, 1983) reminds us of the context in which hermeneutic work is to be evaluated for adequacy by contrasting it to the assumptions of the empiricist school of thought. He states that a hermeneutic science of human beings

> would not be founded on brute data; its primitive data would be readings of meanings, and its object would have the [following] properties . . . : (1) *meanings which are partially constituted by* self-definitions, which are in this sense *already interpretations*, and (2) meanings which can be *re-expressed* or made *explicit*. (p. 133–134)

The subject may be a society or community, but the intersubjective meanings embody a certain self-definition, a vision of the agent and his or her society, which is that of the society or community. The fusion of perspectives of the individual and his or her society is reflected in the interpretative act. This characteristic of hermeneutic data leads us into the question of generalizability.

Generalizability

Gadamer's (1980) achievement of the fusion of horizons between the interpreter's past and present and between the parts and the whole of a text represents an epistemological as well as ontological move out of the particular, historical moment to an "overall *single* horizon in which human life lives" (p. 108). Gadamer talks about this as an elevation to a higher generality, above one's own and the other's particularity. He also talks of the hermeneutic universal. He does not hold as possible the attainment of absolute knowledge. Rather, even the universal nature of knowledge, objectivity, and truth imply historical relativity. However, hermeneutic knowledge as meant by Gadamer at times appears to be an ontological truth similar to Max Scheler's (1962) "ideal essences." As such, this knowledge can only be more or less grasped approximately by persons at different periods, bound as they are to the finite conditions of their lives.

Validity

Gadamer claims that scientism itself it not sufficient to reveal truth. Although Gadamer is unclear about the specifics of how one is to validate claims to truth, his work points us in the direction of the use of tradition and the past to put in perspective the tendencies in modern thought that neglect or are insensitive to tradition and history. Additionally, Gadamer recommends the use of intersubjectivity and public criteria for the evaluation of claims to truth by the community of interpreters. In effect, a "fusion of horizons" between individual and tradition is the nexus to be evaluated. Gadamer's (1980) hermeneutic theory and interpretative act applied to live discussions is judged to be successful not by its logical rigor but by its effectiveness in bringing the essence of the subject matter to light to the extent that the limited conditions of any discussion permit.

This differs radically from Dilthey's empathic but historical transference, and his objective understanding of meanings which ultimately must be judged by "scientific verification." The particularity of historical knowledge allows Dilthey to legitimately use this type of verification. However, the question of generalizability and universality remains unanswered.

The Procedure for Validation. According to Klemm (1983), the procedure for validation of guesses is ruled more by "a logic of probability" (p. 93) rather than by one of empirical verification. The best reading of a text is judged by the one that can justify its "articulation" of the figurative sense with respect to the objective structure of the literal sense. In addition, it is also the most consistent and deepest of construed ways possible.

According to Klemm (1983), the suggested approach to understanding double meaning (literary and poetic) texts is first "to guess the figurative meaning in a naive reading and then to subject that initial understanding to a validation through explanations" (p. 92). Ultimately, the most probable reading of a text is the one that makes the most sense of details in relation to the whole in the most comprehensive way. This validation process is actually Ricoeur's reformulation of the "hermeneutic circle" inherited from Schleiermacher along what he considered more objective lines. Ricoeur placed the dialogue between the discourse as text and the discourse of the interpreter; discourse is "fixed" by writing. As such, the hermeneutic circle is drawn within the wholly semantical space of text interpretations and not in the psychological space created between the subjectivity of the author and that of the interpreter. This reformulation of the hermeneutic circle sets the stage for "structural analysis" in hermeneutics as a method reconstructed by Ricoeur.

Habermas (in Bernstein, 1983) addresses the issue of validity in evaluating speech acts in hermeneutics. He states that "classifying" and "describing" speech acts presupposes that the interpreter has the ability to "make clear to himself or herself the implicit reasons that enable participants to take the positions that they do take" (p. 182). Habermas advocates the use of the "performative attitude" to achieve validity in the hermeneutic process. That is, the interpreter is to engage in "virtual participation with the person acting" whose validity claim is to be evaluated. The first step is to evaluate *whether* or not a validity claim is made by the acting person and, second, and only sequentially, can the interpreter make an evaluative judgment about the *soundness* of that validity claim.

The performative attitude thus requires the interpreter to know a culture well enough to recognize the conditions and reasons by which certain acts are performed by individuals of that culture, time in history, and individual persuasion. For Habermas (in Bernstein, 1983), the performative attitude is the condition for all understanding "whether it is the understanding that arises among participants in communicative action or that of the social scientist who seeks to understand alien linguistic practices" (p. 183). Habermas is very clear about the need for questions of meaning and questions of validity to be linked always.

Reliability. The ability of an interpreter to return again and again to the same understanding achieved once is possible within hermeneutics, specifically by means of the interplay or dialectic process of the hermeneutic circle. Gadamer's (1975a) fusion of individual and traditional horizons represents an understanding that is derived from the interplay of situation and horizon, person and history, and the parts and the whole of a given text. The history of the interpreter, which is also part of the context, reveals prejudices as well as accuracies. The interplay of all three levels of relationship provides the testing ground for reliability of the process leading to intersubjective agreement among interpreters.

PROBLEMS OF IMPLEMENTING HERMENEUTICS

Obviously, hermeneutics requires considerable facility in a language and some mastery of rhetoric and linguistics. These same skills are prerequisite for successful scholarship in graduate nursing. A problem will exist when individuals do not have adequate reading and writing skills.

The most common error in hermeneutics is to interpret things outside of ourselves by standards and norms of the "critical stance" alone and to ignore the potential understanding derived from the stance of ourselves-in-the-world.[23] For example, the description of a boy seen swimming from a distance and in quantifiable terms is neither hermeneutic nor sufficient for human science. But, retaining this objective description of swimmer and recognizing the familiar strokes as common to your own experience, as well as characteristic of a shared culture (American crawl), with access to the swimmer's perceptions, is a comprehensive as well as hermeneutic approach to understanding this human action.

Akin to the above pitfall is the premature desire to bring closure to an understanding under the guise of *objectivity*. Scientific knowledge of matter of fact is not the goal of hermeneutics. As previously discussed, the goal is understanding.

For example, when the nature of nursing as seen from our lived experience takes on a reality shared by many nurses, then the future of nursing can be projected, created, and anticipated on the basis of hermeneutic understanding. In other words, understanding from a belonging standpoint has equal weight to critical interpretation and scientific self-control.

In addition, it is recommended that "understanding" remain before us as an event of human experience and that the interpreting subject not "preside" over it as to control it. A disposition of receptivity and reflexivity is necessary for the recognition of universal attributes (shared) of human understanding itself, as well as of the phenomenon of concern. It is essential to recognize that the hermeneutic phenomenon encompasses both the alien that we strive to understand and the familiar that we already understand. *Forgetfulness* of this principle violates hermeneutics itself.

In the twentieth century, because the "science of hermeneutics" has almost completely ignored the "reflexive" dimension of understanding, a distorted and one-sided view of understanding and of our relationship to tradition has risen. Reflexivity joins the "far" and the "near," past and present.[24] Bernstein (1983) states it perfectly:

> A false picture is suggested when we think that our task is to leap out of our own linguistic horizon, bracket all our preunderstandings, and enter into a radically different world. Rather the task is always to find the resources within our own horizon, linguistic practices, and experience that can enable us to understand what confronts us as alien. (p. 123)

This is the way that we can "risk" and "test" our prejudices and thereby come to understand what confronts us as well as better understand ourselves. Practical wisdom is reclaimed as a concept that impels us to act from an integral standpoint. Basically, it involves learning from what is alien and different rather than *spurning what is strange*.

Danger of Ethnocentrism in Interpretation

Habermas (in Bernstein, 1983) is aware of the danger of ethnocentrism, of unreflectively imposing alien standards of judgment and thereby missing the point or meaning of a practice among a culture. But his primary thesis is that

> it is an illusion to think that we can escape from this danger by imagining that we can describe alien linguistic practices without determining the validity claims that are implicitly made in speech acts. (p. 183)

Determining validity claims is a condition for all understanding whether it arises among participants in communicative action or that of the social scientist seeking to understand alien linguistic practices. To make such an evaluation requires the "performative attitude" of the interpreter or his or her participation in a process of mutual understanding. This requirement may be difficult for some to accomplish. The quality and accuracy of the interpretation is, therefore, dependent upon this process.

Integrating Qualitative and Quantitative Approaches

If one defines quantitative strategies as inquiry leading to "explanation" in science and art and defines qualitative strategies as leading to "understanding" in science and art, then Ricoeur's (1981) hermeneutic theory of interpretation can provide nursing with a promising framework for integrating this seeming dichotomy. Insufficient precision in discussions over quantitative/qualitative distinctions has stalemated our progress. Ricoeur's precise reasoning can be illuminating from a hermeneutic standpoint.

Explanation. Explanation pertains to the analysis of the objective sense of "texts" as a structural work. "Meaningful action" as a focus also exhibits structures like a text which can be analyzed and, therefore, explained from a quantitative approach.

Understanding. In contrast, understanding is not discovered solely from looking at the structured aspects of the text or meaningful action, but rather is refined beyond the structured text to some extralingual reality. This reality can either be inner, outer or spiritual reality within a possible world that we might inhabit. This means a world we can create as well as reconstruct. For example, beyond the text in front of you, understanding can refer to memories, perceptions or anticipations for the future. Thus, the connection between these worlds involves comprehending them in relationship to your own horizon, as well as to the horizon of the person expressing them in written form, speech or meaningful action. Understanding, like comprehension, in reading skills represents an instance akin to the qualitative as well as the quantitative research goal. Accordingly, Ricoeur's (1981) reconciliation of explanation and understanding through the hermeneutics of interpretation gives us a plausible framework for integrating qualitative and quantitative research methods. The key is to recognize that the "evidence" required by each approach is different and thus employs different means of assessing and validating; however, all derive from the same phenomena under study.

The Limits of Structural Analysis. Structural analysis is a strategy used to obtain the objective sense of a written sentence or written text. The syntax of language and the logic of statements are explored. However, the limitation of structural analysis is its inability to interpret what the primary author intended from an historical and cultural context. Only the structure of the language can be addressed.

Speech adds real references in the world to ideal sense, whereas structural analysis excludes "real references." Spoken language, choice, and actualization remain outside the perspective of structural linguistics.

Ricoeur (1981) recognized the strength of structural analysis in its capacity to highlight the importance of arrangement of linguistic elements. However, he voices a number of misgivings. These include: (1) lack of reflexivity which leads to *opting for syntax rather than semantics*; to generalization concerning its investigation which *transgresses its own code of rules* (logic), which is limited to particulars; (2) assigning greater importance to arrangement of elements than to their content or thought; and (3) ineffectiveness in examining traditions and history which, according to Bleicher (1980), have a "surplus of meaning" (p. 225); that is, meaning which goes beyond the use and function of the literal expressions.

Therefore, structural analysis should not be used alone as a hermeneutic tool but, in Ricoeur's (1981) terms, is best used when it serves the purpose of linking "naive understanding" and "hermeneutic understanding" in the fullest sense. Naive understanding, which accepts symbols in their surface-meaning, combined with hermeneutic understanding, which carries sense and reference of many possible worlds and horizons, can be accomplished through Ricoeur's rendering of structural analysis.

Ricoeur (1981) provides reasons for his reconstruction. Because man is not transparent to himself, his existence, therefore, has to be understood in this manner: first, through seeking truth and intending to understand; second, by structural analysis of utterances; and, third, through the process of appropriation or making one's own what was alien.

Ricoeur's (1981) structural analysis thus brings into play an *economy and order* that sets limits on the various meanings possible to language and, at the same time, allows *symbolism* to express its significant character. For it is within the context of a whole that symbols articulate their meaning; that is, words require placement in a sentence (context) to express particular meanings. As mentioned elsewhere, the interpretation of a sentence is often shaped by the interpreter's pre-understandings from his or her culture, which is never "meaningless."

Ricoeur (1981) introduced "eiditic" phenomenology from Husserl into hermeneutic interpretation, which recognizes the life-world *Lebenswelt* as the "belongingness" of naive understanding and the *epoché* as the critical instance of distancing through *reflexivity*.

Thus newly constructed, structural analysis provides distancing to clarify what is understood by the interpreter in front of the written text. Thereafter, Ricoeur (1981) attempts to return the subject back into hermeneutics through the process of appropriation. He reaffirms the necessity of regarding language as an event of speech in addition to language as a system of signs which can be decoded.

Rather than serving only a critical function of dissolving "false consciousness" expressed in language, Ricoeur (1981) brings a characteristically idealist hermeneutic thought back into interpretation which emphasizes the communicative importance of language.

THE ROLE OF HERMENEUTICS IN NURSING SCHOLARSHIP AND THEORY DEVELOPMENT

It should be clear at this point that a discussion on hermeneutics is more than a question of method, but rather encompasses all that can be said about nursing as an "active ontology." I would propose that the discipline and practice of nursing is a mode of being that will realize its best expression in metaphorical language because of the multiple levels of meaning and the dialectical nature of our experience as a profession.

Meleis (1987) recently stated that nursing must "move beyond knowing to really understanding" (p. 6). As a discipline, scholars in nursing have demonstrated natural propensities to know through multiple modalities. This diversity and richness directly shapes the kind of knowledge in nursing that will guide practice, education, and research. This multidimensional propensity also suggests that the pursuit of only one overarching theory or of only one epistemology for nursing would be death-dealing for the profession. Multiple ontologies and modalities are essential to a futuristic approach to theory development in nursing.

The universal linguisticality of all human beings is multidisciplinary, multicultural, and multidimensional in all aspects of life. On this basis, hermeneutics illuminates the power of language to shape us as well as to provide a means to express our experiences and meanings. It permeates all efforts to communicate among and across civilizations and most immediately among and across individuals receiving and giving care.

The contributions hermeneutics can make to scholarship and theory development in nursing can first be realized in doctoral education with Socratic discourse and spoken language. Scholarship is a bridge between thought and the world of experience and begins with the refinement of verbal expression in dialogic seminars on a common topic. Specifically, Gadamer (1976) draws upon Plato's dialogues and recommends "live discussion" and playful dialogue to take us to a level of comprehensive understanding. The value of listening as "uncontentious" players in a game of language provides doctoral students the opportunity to proceed not by tangential references, but by the leading question and subsequent questions evoked in class. For example, the discussion proceeds often to puzzlement rather than to a clear answer deduced with cogent reasoning. The process is not one of methodological deduction, but rather the question continues to prevail over the answer and serves to provoke further thought; new thought provokes new questions and brings one to new insights.

Socratic discourse, illuminated further by Gadamer (1976), involves the skill of listening to the speaker and to the context/meaning of the language expressed at any given time. The object is not to identify the illogic or faults of deduction but rather to grasp the new insights provoked by deliberately confounding statements and by new questions.

Lived experience precedes theory in many disciplines and provides a model for others. Relevant to nursing is the fact that hermeneutics and rhetoric both developed out of the practice and use of language. Theory of forms of speech and persuasion developed out of native talent. Thus, the ontological characteristics and lived experience gave rise to theory after some time of reflection on their importance. This is not to say that theory development in hermeneutics proceeds by "induction." Rather, hermeneutics proceeds by mutual participation for the purpose of understanding.

Another reason for interest in rhetoric is for its broader interpretations of truth claims. Rhetoric is an older discipline than hermeneutics and provides the theoretical tools for the art of interpretation. Gadamer (1976) states that rhetoric traditionally has been

> the only advocate of a claim to truth that defends the probable, the "eikos" (verisimile) and that which is convincing to the ordinary reason, against the claim of science to accept as true what can be demonstrated and tested. (p. 24)

It is no less true that scientific progress reigns by its ability to convince and persuade through rhetoric. This ubiquitous quality of rhetoric renders it larger and more independent than science itself; every discipline that desires to be relevant or of practical use to social life is dependent upon rhetoric.

According to Gadamer (1976), Plato's rhetoric, for example, became a task to master the faculty of speaking in such an effectively persuasive way that "the arguments brought forward are always appropriate to the specific receptivity of the souls to which they are directed" (p. 21).

Aristotle's theory of rhetoric fulfills Plato's requirement that "one must have a profound knowledge of the souls of those one wishes to persuade." In other words, speech and soul must be in mutual accommodation. Using Plato's premise, the doctoral student is challenged to listen intently to the speaker's voice as it shifts throughout the class and to mete out his or her own questions in direct relation to the ongoing dialogic conversation of scholars. Thus, rhetoric clearly is more than words, but encompasses the impact of "speaking" in all its immediacy.

Later, application of rhetoric was made to effective writing with emphasis on style and variation of expression. Again, the rules and theory developed out of a practical project guided by native ability to achieve communication with another. Likewise, the art of understanding in hermeneutics did not begin by following theoretical reflection on ways and means, but rather theory was subsequent to "praxis" in both hermeneutics and rhetoric. And, like rhetoric and hermeneutics, the active ontological mode of nursing precedes us in our choices toward theory development.

Rhetoric and Hermeneutics are Complementary

Rhetoric and hermeneutics foreshadow a model of relationship between quantitative and qualitative differences in nursing research. For example, rhetoric and hermeneutics have contrasting points of origin that ultimately make them complementary. Rhetoric attests to a universal characteristic of human beings called "linguisticality," that is, everyone has some capacity for language to express their relationship to the world and to themselves. This gives rhetoric a *positive* point for departure. In contrast, hermeneutics came to flower in the Romantic era as a consequence of the modern dissolution of firm bonds with tradition. According to Gadamer (1976), it represents an ongoing effort to "grasp something vanishing and to hold it up in the light of consciousness" (p. 21). Hermeneutics occurs in the later stages of cultural evolution. Thus, the "history-embracing and history-preserving" element runs deep in hermeneutics. Rhetoric may be said to be "pro-active" and hermeneutics to be "retro-active."

However, in both rhetoric and hermeneutics, a kind of reflection is shared; a meditation about "praxis" is one that is already natural and sophisticated. Nursing scholarship oriented from a practice perspective is also a natural and sophisticated approach, one that is becoming more reflective. Another type of reflection that may be even more relevant to nursing theory development is provided by Ricoeur.

Ricoeur's (1981) transformation of hermeneutics incorporates a type of reflection borrowed from critical social theory which is a means of "emancipation from authority and tradition." Actual and perceived oppression in the past can certainly be a source of conflict and pain in the present and calls for emancipation and freedom. At the system or personal level, understanding and consent are recognized as essential to freedom. The hermeneutic task has developed out of an awareness that mutual understanding has been disturbed and that those involved must search for and find or create it again together.

It is important to note that mutual understanding does not mean static relationship or knowledge achieved once and for all. But understanding is a goal toward which the hermeneutic circle takes us in an ongoing spiral upward, forever being created. Because of the evolutionary nature of humans and the universe, a dialectic of differences and similarities is a universal characteristic of the human attempt to understand and find meaning in life.

Relevance to Nursing

A scholarly approach to the development of theory in nursing from a hermeneutical perspective is probably inherent in all possible approaches because of the universal and required human characteristic of "linguisticality." Adequate interpretation of language is a basic assumption of scholarship. However, theories offer alternative interpretations of language and are extremely beneficial to a discipline with ethical and social responsibility. It would seem highly advisable to choose a hermeneutic perspective (or create one) that has the following preferred characteristics:

1. The hermeneutic interplay unites explanation in science and understanding of hermeneutics to illuminate the nature of nursing's questions.

2. The hermeneutic interplay bridges history, tradition, and original intentions of the author/speaker/actor with the present discourse to increase understanding.

3. The hermeneutic interplay is an ongoing reconciliation of theory and praxis employing sympathetic, critical, and humoristic attitudes.

4. The hermeneutic interplay moves understanding toward emancipation and freedom impelled by rationality and compassion.

5. A "fusion of horizons" between past, present and future, as well as between individuals in separate situations, is the goal of the hermeneutic circle to deepen and broaden understanding through language.

6. A dialectic of belongingness, distanciation, and appropriation may be addressed in a nursing hermeneutic theory of human caring from multiple discourses.

7. Criteria of effective hermeneutics of metaphor may be recognized in the realization of enlarged and deepened understanding of exemplary texts agreed upon intersubjectively over time.

8. The performative attitude and communicative action may be addressed in coming to understand human relationships in practical discourse to increase the possibility of agreement and of normative action.

9. The hermeneutic interplay addresses sensitivity to sexist use of language to enhance the emancipatory role of spoken and written words.

In summary, a hermeneutical approach to the development of nursing theory would be characterized by theories which seek to bridge the personal experiences of nursing (past, present, and future) and the enlarged, deepening understanding of our common impelling motive for existence and purpose. It seems crucial to illuminate through hermeneutics the persistent enduring values and goals of our discipline which empower, emancipate, and impassion human caring and awaken sensitivity to our shared human condition/situation. Respect and skillful use of the power of language is one of our most distinctive human expressions in pursuit of these goals.

The most common use of hermeneutics in the nursing literature is derived from the perspectives of Gadamer, Ricoeur, and Heidegger.

Benner (1984), in *Novice to Expert*, devised an approach from Heidegger's combined with influence from M. Polanyi's personal knowledge and the "Dryfus Model" of learning from the novice to expert competency level. The unit of Benner's analysis is human action as observed by the investigator as well as described by nurses in practice. Benner's approach emphasizes the value of naive, precognitive experience as a source of wisdom upon which other types of knowledge and action can develop.

Smerke (1988) developed hermeneutic strategies from the perspective of Gadamer and Ricoeur. Interview data, literary texts, and art in the form of screen production were used. The outcome was expressed in the form of metaphor to capture the meaning of caring and noncaring behaviors. Davidson (1988) also developed strategies influenced from the perspectives of Gadamer and Ricoeur. The meaning of experience of the environment and its relation to productivity and creativity were accessible to hermeneutical analyses which focused on written language on transcribed tapes and responses to questionnaires. This study had a quantitative and qualitative section and used a design informed by Ricoeur's fusion of both explanation and understanding through a hermeneutics of distanciation and belongingness. The results of the study show the value of this multiple approach; insights and knowledge omitted by one was provided by the other.

Berrey's (1987) hermeneutical study of the lives of eminent women in nursing utilized a strategy influenced by Heidegger's (1962) hermeneutics in *Being and Time*, specifically the ontological mode of being of understanding itself, as well as feminist perspectives on the use of language in science and life in general (Fiorenza, 1984). The question of intention of the author conveyed through the context and structure of language is emphasized in this study and leads the way to an integral hermeneutic most accommodating to phenomena of concern to the discipline and profession of nursing.

Allen (1985) has developed a model of hermeneutic analysis from a critical social theorist point of view, drawing upon Habermas and Ricoeur, as well as feminist perspectives in science. The goal of such research is to bridge the subtle levels of understanding through attention to language meanings with the emancipatory view of efficacy in human action from a critical social concern for the well-being of society. Again, the combination of methods of inquiry highlight the benefits beyond any singular approach.

FOOTNOTES

[1]Schleiermacher's "Theory of the Art of Understanding" represents a masterful use of Romantic as well as Critical Philosophy and can be traced down through the tradition that followed.

[2]The reflexive aspect of hermeneutics was totally ignored, which is surprising because Dilthey based the continuity of historicity originally on Husserl's principle of inner-time consciousness, which Husserl intended to be reflexive.

[3]This ontological position was a move against Neo-Kantian idealism and the earlier works of Edmund Husserl (1859–1938), founder of the Phenomenological Movement. Gadamer and Heidegger's approach challenged the programme of Husserl. Historically, it became clear that their hermeneutical critique toppled the most idealistic form of phenomenology offered by Husserl in his earliest writings. However, his later writings and phenomenology as such is recognized to have great affinity with hermeneutics. For example, hermeneutics shares with phenomenology both the assumption that the question of meaning is primary, and the thesis that the source of meaning is anterior to language, as in the lived world.

[4]Philosophical hermeneutics was viewed by Gadamer through the influence of Plato, Aristotle, Hegel, and Heidegger. His hermeneutic method was that of Heidegger in the phenomenological tradition: however, Gadamer drew upon themes implicit in Heidegger which he then developed in novel ways.

[5]According to Ricoeur (1981), Gadamer moved Heidegger's hermeneutical thinking away from ontology and towards epistemological problems. Gadamer attempts, thereby, to overcome posed oppositions inherited from the Enlightenment, such as those between reason and tradition, reason and prejudice, and reason and authority. His answer combines ontological and epistemological perspectives when he states (in Bernstein, 1983):

> Reason is not a faculty or capacity that can free itself from its historical context and horizons. Reason is historical or situated reason which gains its distinctive power always within a living tradition. (p. 37)

Gadamer carefully critiques the historic philosophical struggles between Romanticism and the Enlightenment, Dilthey against positivism, and Heidegger against Neo-Kantianism, before he presents his own positions.

[6]A synthesis of ontological positions related to "being-in-the-world," a notion borrowed and extended from Heidegger (1962), is seen as the source of understanding itself: "Understanding is man's primordial mode of being." Gadamer (1975a,b; 1976; 1980) extends this notion to the interpreter of human action in an effort toward understanding.

[7]For example, Gadamer (1975) explains that the use of the word "praxis" is Aristotelian in the sense that it is practical reason, knowledge, and action together that forms "the methodological model for self-understanding of the human sciences" (p. 107). Gadamer also states that this definition is very different from the modern use of the word, which has been "deformed by degrading practical reason to technical control" (p. 312).

[8]The affinity between the phenomenological and hermeneutical traditions provides the philosophical basis for Paul Ricoeur's work.

[9]This breakthrough, which appears only in the later works of Ricoeur, emphasizes hermeneutic method explicitly. This marks a shift away from the phenomenological emphasis of his earlier works, which focused on hidden meanings of symbols, to the critical instance highlighted and created by his later works, where reference and meaning "in front of the text" becomes the focus. Above all, use of distanciation made it possible and necessary for Ricoeur (1981) to examine the presuppositions of hermeneutics themselves.

Notably, the "critical instance" is seen to be necessary as a reflective and "objectifying" event within the hermeneutic perspective. Instead of being opposed to the "belonging instance of interpretation," the "critical instance" joins belonging in the spiraling dance moving toward greater understanding. The change in Ricoeur's (1981) method is closely connected to a displacement of the initial object of investigation; the immediate focus is no longer the intentional objects of subjective processes, or even the symbolic expressions of personal experiences, as in phenomenology, but becomes the entire domain of written discourse of texts and analogues of texts. The ultimate work of Ricoeur's life is his poetics of the will. Ricoeur's emphasis on "the will" is a justification of hermeneutics by a necessary seeking of "reflective thought"; consciousness alone is not enough for understanding.

Ricoeur's (1981) thought has been bold and broad, which is not surprising when one casts an eye over the contributions of the many intellectual traditions which informed his work: hermeneutics and phenomenology, analytic philosophy, structuralism, and critical theory all have had their mark. However, these contributions were molded into a perspective by

Ricoeur which is original and unique. In addition, Ricoeur is a philosopher in the classical sense, a thinker who turns his attention to diverse domains and who expresses his views on issues of social, political, and intellectual concern.

[10]From his perspective, neither Marx's critique of ideology nor the critical theory of the older Frankfurt thinkers, such as Max Horkheimer, provides an adequate answer to this foundational question.

[11]Habermas was aware of the dialectic of the Enlightenment, recognized its dark side, but was convinced there was still a way of redeeming, reconstructing, and rationally defending the "emancipatory aspirations of the Enlightenment." Ultimately, this would necessitate a call for autonomy and concrete freedom embracing all of humankind (Bernstein, 1983).

The difference between Gadamer and Habermas is not only the span of 30 years that separates them but the historical circumstances that had decisive influence on their intellectual development. As experienced before World War I and II, and in line with German Romanticism, Gadamer saw the world as "continuous." As lived after World War I and II, and with a memory of destruction and separation of immense and immediate consequences, Habermas saw the world as "discontinuous."

[12]The most current and accurate reading of Schleiermacher's works is the translation and versions by Kimmerle (1977). That is, the author's earlier as well as later works are presented and, most importantly, reflect both the Romantic genius and the critical approach to interpretation and understanding. Earlier critiques of Schleiermacher by Dilthey, Gadamer, Ricoeur, and Habermas took into account only the psychological aspect of his earlier works; therefore, their reconstructions of hermeneutics reflect a dirth of critical themes in Schleiermacher's hermeneutics. Nursing researchers will benefit from revisiting Schleiermacher in the Kimmerle renditions for a more balanced view.

[13]Dilthey drew upon Husserl's definition of "expression" as it appeared in his *Logical Investigations* of 1900 to secure the objectivity of written expressions of life in historical texts. Essentially, expressions were "speech acts and similar signs" which signify something; an objectivity, to which it refers. Ultimately, Dilthey (in Klemm, 1983) stated "expressions of life in texts are to be grasped as referring both to the objective cultural spheres and to the inner power of the individual" (p. 25).

[14]Heidegger disregards the previous conception of being as "supreme being as the sum total of positive predicates." *Dasein* is the place to begin because self-knowledge is enough to tell us that we as being are "concerned about being"; therefore, we (*Dasein*) understand ourselves in our

being in some "manner and explicitness." Heidegger (1962) asserts that "understanding of being is itself a defining characteristic of the being of *Dasein*."

[15]That is, through a hermeneutic interplay between the reference (expressions of being) and sense (concern about being) a fundamental ontology can be developed.

[16]Heidegger does not provide an epistemology for understanding "understanding," but rather conceives of "ontology" as a hermeneutic of *Dasein* based on his belief that *Dasein* has the character of a sign itself pointing to a "sense" or meaning. The hermeneutic circle of understanding is applied to the relation between *sign* and *sense* of *Dasein* itself. The two are to be reconciled. It is a reflective hermeneutic process directed at the being of *Dasein* from an "*a priori*" nonexperiential, speculative world view.

However, Heidegger failed to arrive at an interpretation of the meaning of being due to false assumptions about temporality. He had hoped to take the "being of *Dasein*" as a sign pointing to "being as such" as the leading meaning of the various modes of being. This was the reason for calling his work a hermeneutic of *Dasein*. But much to his dismay, according to Klemm (1983), the sign pointing to being still "remains without interpretation" (p. 44).

[17]Further, according to Bernstein (1983), the notion of freedom appropriated from Plato, Hegel, and Aristotle drives Gadamer's pursuit of understanding for practical purposes; he sees hermeneutics, after Aristotle, as a practical philosophy. He accepts Hegel's principles of freedom as "a freedom that is realized only when there is authentic mutual 'recognition' among individuals" (p. 163).

[18]For Gadamer (1975a), language is the medium of the act of appropriation within the "fusion of horizons."

[19]Ricoeur likens the initial "guess" to what Schleiermacher called the "divinatory" aspect of reading. And as with Schleiermacher, the skilled reader is aware that he or she will submit the first reading to a "structural" explanation as corrective. Thus, what is to be guessed is the meaning of the text as a whole, the meaning of the text as an individual, and the meaning of the text as a product of style. The latter involves determining which horizons of potential meaning are actualized. This actualization is said to come about through the "metaphoric-symbolic style of the text," a product of Ricoeur's in hermeneutics.

[20]Ricoeur does not limit his approach to French structuralist ideology. This ideology, which was learned from Levi-Strauss, concentrates on narrative form for underlying codes which constitute the single meaning

of the text. Rather, for Ricoeur (1981), a range of possible world references representing patterns of interconnections in the text can be displayed as "spectator world, world recalled, auditory world, world imagined, etc.," (p. 94). Also, the modes of awareness of the world can be isolated as sight, memory, sound, imagination, etc. Lastly, through reflexivity upon language, the kinds of self can be isolated as spectator-self, self-remembering-self, hearkening-self, etc. Ultimately, Ricouer does not find structural analysis à la Levi-Strauss sufficient for his hermeneutics.

[21]Ricoeur's (1981) interpretation of the act of reflection contrasts with that described by Husserl for phenomenology, which holds that "immediate consciousness of the world or intellectual intuition (grasping) is possible of essences before deliberate thematizing of external manifestations of the life-world" (p. 81).

[22]Here explanation and understanding are reconciled through the mediation of structural analysis by linking pre-understandings with hermeneutic interpretation in this three-fold approach.

[23]The balance between these two sources of understanding engages both Romantic genius and the Critical theorist's point of view as proposed first by Schleiermacher.

[24]Examples of this tendency to ignore reflexivity in the use of hermeneutics is seen in the works of Dilthey's historical hermeneutics. Reflexivity is not incompatible with historical data but Dilthey lost this dimension due to an overreliance on the natural science method and adherence to a seventeenth-century view of objectivity.

In contrast, Gadamer defines the "hermeneutic situation" to include the historicity of the interpreter and, by doing so, recognized the positive contribution of "prejudice" and "bias" to understanding. Moreover, these two historical attributes of an interpreter provide the context and horizon against which understanding develops and is tested through the interplay of interpretation.

REFERENCES

Allen, D. (1985). Nursing research and social control: Alternative models of science that emphasize understanding and emancipation. *Image, 17* (2), 59–65.

Allen, D., Benner, P., & Diekelmann, N. L. (1986). Three paradigms for nursing research: Methodological implications. In P. Chinn (Ed.), *Nursing research methodology* (pp. 23–38). Salem, MA: Aspen Publishers, Inc.

Benhabib, S., & Cornell, D. (Eds.). (1987). *Feminism as critique: On the politics of gender.* Minneapolis: University of Minnesota Press.

Benner, P. (1984). *From novice to expert*. Menlo Park, CA: Addison-Wesley.

Benoliel, J. Q. (1987). Response to Schultz. *Scholarly Inquiry for Nursing Practice*, *1*(2), p. 147–152.

Bernstein, R. (1983). *Beyond objectivism and relativism*. Philadelphia: University of Pennsylvania Press.

Berrey, E. (1987). *Researching the lives of eminent women in nursing*. Unpublished dissertation. Ann Arbor, MI: University Microfilm International, Case Western Reserve University.

Bleicher, J. (1980). *Contemporary hermeneutics. Hermeneutics as method, philosophy and critique*. London: Routledge and Kegan Paul.

Bleicher, J. (1982). *The hermeneutic imagination*. London: Routledge & Kegan Paul.

Chinn, P. (1986). *Nursing research methodology*. Rockville, MD: Aspen Publishers, Inc.

Davidson, A. (1988). *Human/environment relationship patterns at work*. Unpublished dissertation. Boulder, CO: University Microfilm International, University of Colorado.

Dilthey, W. (1927). *Der aufbau der Geschichtlichen welt in den geisteswissenschaften, vol.7 of Wilhelm Dilthey's gessamelte schriften*. Leipzig and Berlin: B. G. Teubner.

Dilthey, W. (1972). The rise of hermeneutics. (F. Jameson, Trans.), *New literary history 3*.

Dilthey, W. (1975). *Philosophy of the human sciences* (R. Makreel, Trans.). Princeton, NJ: Princeton University Press.

Dilthey, W. (1976). The development of hermeneutics. In H. P. Richman (Ed. and Trans.), *Selected writings*. Cambridge, MA: Cambridge University Press.

Fiorenza, E. S. (1984). *Bread not stone: The challenges of feminist biblical interpretations*. Boston: Beacon Press.

Frei, H. (1974). *The eclipse of biblical narrative*. New Haven: Yale University Press.

Gadamer, H. G. (1975a). *Truth and method* (B. Garrett & J. Cumming, Trans. & Eds.). New York: Seabury Press.

Gadamer, H. G. (1975b). Hermeneutics and social science. *Cultural Hermeneutics*, *2*, 312.

Gadamer, H. G. (1976). *Philosophical hermeneutics* (D. E. Linge, Trans.). Berkeley: University of California Press.

Gadamer, H. G. (1979). The problem of historical consciousness. In P. Rabinow & W. M. Sullivan (Eds.), *Interpretative social sciences: A reader*. Berkeley: University of California Press.

Gadamer, H. G. (1980). *Dialogue and dialectic: Eight hermeneutical studies on Plato* (P. C. Smith, Trans.). New Haven: Yale University Press.

Geertz, C. (1979). From the native's point of view: On the nature of anthropological understanding. In Rabinow & Sullivan (Eds.), *Interpretative social science: A reader*. Berkeley: University of California Press.

Geertz, C. (1979). Deep play: Notes on the Balinese cockfight. In Rabinow & Sullivan (Eds.), *Interpretative social science: A reader*. Berkeley: University of California Press.

Gortner, S., & Schultz, P. R. (1988). Approaches to nursing science methods. *Image, 20*(1), p. 22–24.

Grooten, J. (Ed.). (1957). *The new encyclopedia of philosophy*. New York: Philosophical Library Publishers. (Reprinted in 1972)

Habermas, J. (1971). *Knowledge and human interest* (J. J. Shapiro, Trans.). Boston: Beacon Press.

Habermas, J. (1973). *Theory and practice* (J. Viertel, Trans.). Boston: Beacon Press.

Habermas, J. (1975). *Legitimation crisis* (T. McCarthy, Trans.). Boston: Beacon Press.

Habermas, J. (1979). *Communication and the evolution of society*. (T. McCarthy, Trans.). Boston: Beacon Press.

Heelan, P. (1982). Hermeneutical realism and scientific observation. *Philosophy of Science Association, 1*, 77–87.

Heidegger, M. (1962). *Being and time* (J. Macquarrie & E. Robinson, Trans.). New York: Harper and Row.

Klemm, D. (1983). *The hermeneutical theory of Paul Ricoeur*. East Brunswick, NJ: Associated University Press, Inc.

Meleis, A. A. (1987). Epistemology: The nature of knowledge. *Proceedings of the Fourth Nursing Science Colloquium. Strategies for Theory Development in Nursing, IV* (pp. 5–18). Boston: Boston University School of Nursing.

Palmer, R. (1969). *Hermeneutics: Interpretation theory in Schleiermacher, Dilthey, Heidegger, and Gadamer*. Evanston, IL: Northwestern University Press.

Rabinow, P., & Sullivan, W. M. (Eds.). (1979). *Interpretative social sciences: A reader*. Berkeley: University of California Press.

Reeder, F. (1984). *Nursing research, holism and philosophy of science: Points of congruence between M. E. Rogers and E. Husserl*. Ann Arbor, MI: Microfilm International, University of Colorado.

Ricoeur, P. (1967). *Husserl: An analysis of his phenomenology*. Evanston, IL: Northwestern University Press.

Ricoeur, P. (1981). *Hermeneutics and the human sciences*. Cambridge: Cambridge University Press.

Scheler, M. (1962). *Man's place in nature*. (H. Meyeroff, Trans.). New York: The Noon Day Press.

Schleiermacher, F. (1977). *Hermeneutics: The handwritten manuscripts* (H. Kimmerle, Ed. and J. Duke & J. Forstman, Trans.). Atlanta, GA: Scholars Press.

Schultz, P. R. (1987a). Toward holistic inquiry in nursing: A proposal for synthesis of patterns and methods. *Scholarly Inquiry for Nursing Practice: An International Journal, 1*(2), p. 135–146.

Schultz, P. R. (1987b). When the client is more than one: Extending the foundational concept of 'person.' *Advances in Nursing Science, 10*(2), pp. 71–86.

Shapiro, G., & Sica, A. (Eds). (1984). *Hermeneutics: Questions and prospects.* Amherst: The University of Massachusetts Press.

Smerke, J. (1988). *The discovery and creation of the meaning of human caring through the development of a guide to the caring literature.* Unpublished dissertation. Ann Arbor, MI: Microfilm International, University of Colorado.

Taylor, C. (1979). Interpretation and the sciences of man. In Rabinow & Sullivan (Eds.), *Interpretative social science: A reader.* Berkeley: University of California Press.

Thompson, J. L. (1987). Critical scholarship: The critique of domination in nursing. *Advances in Nursing Science, 10*(1), 27–38.

Tracy, D. (1987). *Plurality and ambiguity: Hermeneutics, religion, hope.* San Francisco: Harper & Row.

Wilkie, D. (1987). Hermeneutic research method congruent with the nursing perspective. In S. R. Gortner (Ed.), *Nursing science methods: A reader.* San Francisco: Regents, University of California.